T0093199

Humane Professions

In this compelling history of the co-ordinated, transnational defence of medical experimentation in the nineteenth and early twentieth centuries, Rob Boddice explores the experience of vivisection as humanitarian practice. He captures the rise of the professional and specialist medical scientist, whose métier was animal experimentation and whose guiding principle was 'humanity' or the reduction of the aggregate of suffering in the world. He also highlights the rhetorical rehearsal of scientific practices as humane and humanitarian and connects these often defensive professions to meaningful changes in the experience of doing science. *Humane Professions* examines the strategies employed by the medical establishment to try to cement an idea in the public consciousness: that the blood spilt in medical laboratories served a far-reaching human good.

Rob Boddice is currently a senior research fellow at the Academy of Finland Centre of Excellence in the History of Experiences, Tampere University, Finland. He is an internationally renowned scholar in the histories of emotions, science and medicine. His previous volumes include *The Science of Sympathy* (2016), *Pain: A Very Short Introduction* (2017), *The History of Emotions* (2018) and *A History of Feelings* (2019). This is his tenth book.

Humane Professions

The Defence of Experimental Medicine,
1876–1914

Rob Boddice

Tampere University

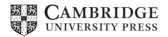
CAMBRIDGE
UNIVERSITY PRESS

CAMBRIDGE
UNIVERSITY PRESS

University Printing House, Cambridge CB2 8BS, United Kingdom

One Liberty Plaza, 20th Floor, New York, NY 10006, USA

477 Williamstown Road, Port Melbourne, VIC 3207, Australia

314–321, 3rd Floor, Plot 3, Splendor Forum, Jasola District Centre, New Delhi – 110025, India

79 Anson Road, #06–04/06, Singapore 079906

Cambridge University Press is part of the University of Cambridge.

It furthers the University's mission by disseminating knowledge in the pursuit of education, learning, and research at the highest international levels of excellence.

www.cambridge.org
Information on this title: www.cambridge.org/9781108490092
DOI: 10.1017/9781108780087

First published 2021

A catalogue record for this publication is available from the British Library.

ISBN 978-1-108-49009-2 Hardback

For Wolfgang Behringer

Contents

Illustrations

Acknowledgements

This book has been more than ten years in the making. It began with a year's postdoctoral fellowship at the Department of the History of Science at Harvard in 2009–10. The research I did that year at the Countway Library of Medicine in Boston was foundational for what became a much broader and international archival search.

For feedback on work in progress, thanks to the history department at the University of Saskatchewan, and Rob Englebert in particular; the attendees of the European Social Science History Conference at Belfast in 2018, on a panel organized by Pilar Leòn Sanz; the participants of the Society for the Social History of Medicine conference in Liverpool, 2018, and especially my co-presenters, Leticia Fernández-Fontecha Rumeu, Dolorès Martin Moruno and Gian Marco Vidor; Will Abberley and the participants of the Emotional Knowledge workshop at the University of Sussex, 2018; the research seminar of the Department of Social Studies of Medicine at McGill, and David Wright, Margaret Lock, Thomas Schlich and George Weisz, in particular, for their insightful questions (George Weisz and Thomas Schlich are owed extra gratitude for their material help in getting this project off the ground in the first place); the Explorations in the Medical Humanities workshop at Columbia University, 2019, particularly the organizers Arden Hegele and Rishi Goyal, and also Thomas Dodman, who provided commentary; the participants of the Canadian Society for the History of Medicine congress in Vancouver, 2019, and my co-presenter on that occasion, Cynthia Tang; and the participants of the Northeast Conference on British Studies in Montreal, 2019.

Invaluable institutional and administrative support has come from Thomas Weitner and Andrea Ladányi in Berlin, who have relieved me of enormous headaches in the process of repeatedly working across international borders. The book would have been impossible without the trust given and freedom afforded by Martin Lücke in Berlin. I reserve special mention for the long-term help and support of Christina Becher, sadly lost to us.

Rine Veith provided an essential piece of the research puzzle from the National Archives in London, as did Mike Esbester from the Bodleian Library in Oxford. To them and to Tom Rosenbaum, Lee Hiltzik (Rockefeller Archive Center) and Stephen Novak (Columbia), many thanks. Mary Yearl and Bozena Latincic at the Osler Library in Montreal greatly facilitated the core contextual work, as part of the curation of the exhibition 'Experiment, Experience, Expertise', which was first blighted by a fire at the Osler Library and was latterly blighted by COVID-19. With any luck, the exhibition will actually take place in 2021. Jan Casper helped enormously to sort and make sense of German primary materials. Elsbeth Heaman wondered aloud what I would make of the MRC, thus alerting me to the fact that I should indeed make something of the MRC. Greg Fisher and Paola Russo provided warmth, sympathy and nourishment, both culinary and human. Inge Rumler Olsen and Gerald W. Olsen provided essential support, making both living and working possible when it otherwise would not be.

The project was funded by the European Union's Horizon 2020 research and innovation programme under the Marie Sklodowska-Curie grant agreement no. 742470 and was completed at the Department of Social Studies of Medicine, McGill University; the Department of History and Cultural Studies, Freie Universität Berlin; and the Academy of Finland Centre of Excellence in the History of Experiences, Tampere University.

Chapter 2 employs material (largely revised, excerpted and expanded) from 'German Methods, English Morals: Physiological Networks and the Question of Callousness, c. 1870–1881', in *Anglo-German Scholarly Networks in the Long Nineteenth Century*, ed. Heather Ellis and Ulrike Kirchberger (Leiden: Brill, 2014). Re-used with permission.

The book is dedicated to Wolfgang Behringer, who set me on a path between 2001 and 2003 that was defined by his intellectual curiosity, constant writing and the assumption that great things would happen. Such profound positivity is rare in academia, and I feel blessed to have been touched by his inspiration.

The work stands indebted to Tony Morris for getting the book over the start line at Cambridge University Press; to Lucy Rhymer for believing in the book's promise; to Liz Friend-Smith for reaching out to me in Belfast and for putting the proposal in Lucy's hands; and to Stephanie Olsen for sharing every minute of the writing process, as she has with every other book. And finally, a big thank-you to Sébastien, for endless cheer between winter lands, whether in lockdown or at 35,000 feet.

Introduction: Experior

Humanity. What is that? What does it mean? It is, in a simple sense, a marker of species. But then, I have spent almost two decades thinking and writing about the history of the ways in which this species has defined itself, marked itself out as distinct or superior, drawn lines of exclusion at the expense of other animals and, often, other beings which sought to lay equal claim to the name 'human'.[1] In a more complex yet narrower sense, 'humanity' encompasses a set of practices comprising dynamically related clusters of experiences, emotions, sensations and thought, that *certain* humans have and do that define them, and only them, as such. Since the Enlightenment at least, 'humanity' has functioned as a synonym, more or less, of sympathy, compassion and pity and, much more recently, of empathy and altruism. It has marked a passional disposition of regard for others, whether human or other animal, with accompanying acts of succour for their suffering. It was definitive of that other Enlightenment master category, *civilization*. In this narrow sense it should be immediately clear that 'humanity' is political: its practice implies an embodied or an embrained quality limited to those who know (1) how to claim it; (2) how to dispense it; (3) how to discriminate among those deserving of it, or not; and (4) of its social value and function. This book, in its broadest terms, is about a breach in this compound knowledge, in the decades either side of 1900.

What I mean by this is that the meaning and experience of 'humanity', including its rhetorical construction, its emotional qualities and its associated activities, changed over time. At the moment of rupture, when

---

[1] Rob Boddice, 'The Moral Status of Animals and the Historical Human Cachet', *JAC: A Journal of Rhetoric, Culture and Politics*, 30:3–4 (2010); Rob Boddice, 'The End of Anthropocentrism', in *Anthropocentrism: Humans, Animals, Environments*, ed. Rob Boddice (Leiden: Brill, 2011); 'The Historical Animal Mind: "Sagacity" in Nineteenth-Century Britain', in *Experiencing Animals: Encounters between Animal and Human Minds*, ed. Robert W. Mitchell and Julie Smith (New York: Columbia University Press, 2012); 'Bestiality in a Time of Smallpox: Dr Jenner and the "Modern Chimera"', in *Exploring Animal Encounters: Philosophical, Cultural and Historical Perspectives*, ed. Dominik Ohrem and Matthew Calarco (London: Palgrave, 2018).

different versions of 'humanity' might be said to have been in competition, it seemed that civilization itself was at stake: on the one side, a prevailing understanding of humanity as Christian compassion; on the other side, an increasingly complex 'faith' in scientific knowledge and its production, coupled with the practices of that production. In fact, the book is only really concerned with this other side. Many before me have attempted to capture the history of the former. But the equation of scientific knowledge production to a practice of humanity is largely uncharted territory. As such, the book is a contribution to a growing body of work on the history of humanitarianism. What it shares with that body of work is a focus on the particular formation of an affective disposition and an accompanying set of practices, but it is at a stage of remove from the historiography's specific foci on nursing, explicitly humanitarian institutions such as the Red Cross and their protocols, philanthropy, war relief or abolition.[2] What is distinct about the humanitarianism in this case is that the cultivated feeling was experienced without having recourse to the *direct* experience of assisting or relieving other humans, and that there was a perceived need to justify and defend this kind of humanitarianism from its detractors who saw it precisely as the opposite of humane. Vivisection seems, on the face of it, to sit at odds with the rise of animal welfare as part of a narrative of humanitarian expansion in the nineteenth century, and accordingly the arguments of medical scientists and their allies with respect to the humanitarianism of experimentation have been essentially overlooked.[3]

---

[2] See Rebecca Gill, *Calculating Compassion: Humanity and Relief in War, Britain, 1870–1914* (Manchester: Manchester University Press, 2013); Karen Halttunen, 'Humanitarianism and the Pornography of Pain in Anglo-American Culture', *American Historical Review*, 100 (1995): 303–34; Thomas L. Haskell, 'Capitalism and the Origins of the Humanitarian Sensibility', parts I and II, *American Historical Review*, 90 (1985): 339–61, 547–66; John Hutchison, *Champions of Charity: War and the Rise of the Red Cross* (Boulder, CO: Westview Press, 1996); Dolores Martín Moruno, Brenda Lynn Edgar and Marie Leyder, 'Feminist Perspectives on the History of Humanitarian Relief (1870–1945)', *Medicine, Conflict and Survival*, 36 (2020): 2–18; Silvia Salvatici, *A History of Humanitarianism, 1755–1989: In the Name of Others* (Manchester: Manchester University Press, 2019); Bertrand Taithe, '"Cold Calculation in the Faces of Horrors?" Pity, Compassion and the Making of Humanitarian Protocols', in *Medicine, Emotion and Disease, 1700–1950*, ed. Fay Bound Alberti (Houdmills, UK: Palgrave, 2006), 79–99; Bertand Taithe and John Borton, 'History, Memory and "Lessons Learnt" from Humanitarian Practitioners', *European Review of History: Revue européenne d'histoire*, 23 (2016): 210–24.

[3] I have emphasized elsewhere the historiographical tendency to assume the historical position of antivivisectionists and the tendency to accept without criticism that animal-loving vivisectors, or experimenting humanitarians, must have had split personalities or, at best, conflicted emotions, Jekyll-and-Hyde-like. For discursion on this point, see Rob Boddice, *The Science of Sympathy: Morality, Evolution and Victorian Civilization* (Urbana: University of Illinois Press, 2016), 75–92, and the following for explicit

Hence this book's title, *Humane Professions*. It conjures with a variety of meanings that aim to capture, on the one hand, the rise of the professional and specialist medical scientist, whose métier was animal experimentation, and whose guiding principle was 'humanity', or the reduction of the aggregate of suffering in the world. On the other hand, it highlights the rhetorical rehearsal – the discursive *profession* – of scientific practices as humane and humanitarian, and connects these often defensive professions, in turn, to meaningful changes in the experience of doing science. For decades, beginning in the 1870s, there was significant emotion work on the part of medical researchers to internalize the practices of animal experimentation as practices of sympathy, to justify a certain affective coolness that was necessary for laboratory work and transform it into a humanitarian medical masculinity. This I have characterized as a kind of conscious callousness – William Osler famously put it under the head of *aequanimitas*, or imperturbability – that suspended immediate aesthetic responses to the sight of suffering and projected forwards to the far-reaching goods that such work seemed to promise.[4] This emotion work was, for many, essential to the formation of the scientific self: a way of justifying means by probable ends, and a way of translating horror into heart work. Routine practices of vivisection became both banal to the practitioner as well as being projected as medical expressions of a well-intentioned mercy.

The book is therefore a logical sequel to my 2016 book, *The Science of Sympathy*, which demonstrated a connection between new ideas of sympathy as 'social glue' that originated in Charles Darwin's (1809–82) *Descent of Man*, and scientific practices of this new sympathy in vivisection, vaccination and eugenics.[5] To the extent that *Science of Sympathy* discussed vivisection and physiology, there is some overlap here, especially in Chapter 1. But my focus in that book was principally on Britain and, concerning vivisection, was limited to the 1870s and 1880s. I use

---

examples: Patrizia Guarnieri, 'Mortitz Schiff (1823–96): Experimental Physiology and Noble Sentiment in Florence', in *Vivisection in Historical Perspective*, ed. Rupke, 106; Hilda Kean, '"The Smooth Cool Men of Science": The Feminist and Socialist Response to Vivisection', *History Workshop Journal*, 40 (1995): 19, 23; Stewart Richards, 'Drawing the Life-Blood of Physiology: Vivisection and the Physiologists' Dilemma, 1870–1900', *Annals of Science*, 43 (1996): 31, 47–80; Paul S. White, 'The Experimental Animal in Victorian Britain', in *Thinking with Animals: New Perspectives on Anthropomorphism*, ed. Lorraine Daston and Gregg Mitman (New York: Columbia University Press, 2005), 62, 74; Paul S. White, 'Sympathy under the Knife: Experimentation and Emotion in Late Victorian Medicine', in *Medicine, Emotion and Disease, 1700–1950*, ed. Fay Bound Alberti (Houndmills, UK: Palgrave, 2006); Paul S. White, 'Darwin Wept: Science and the Sentimental Subject', *Journal of Victorian Culture*, 16 (2011): 195–213.

[4] See Boddice, *Science of Sympathy, passim*. For Osler, see Chapter 2. For physiologists, see Chapters 3 and 4.

[5] Boddice, *Science of Sympathy*.

this as a starting point in *Humane Professions*, expanding the scope to include the period up until the First World War, and expanding the range to include Germany and the USA. It should perhaps be stated explicitly at the outset, therefore, that while the historiography concerning antivivisection has foregrounded questions of animal welfare, of the relative status of animals in relation to humans, and of the nature and politics of pain, here I allude to these things only tangentially, to the extent that they played a part in the defence of experimental medicine or the experience of experimental medicine, either as discourses or practices of humanity.

Conflagration

Scene: New York, 1911. Lower East Side tenement. Context: epidemic diseases, diphtheria, viral meningitis. Metaphor: fire.

As the flames of disease threatened to raze civilization, the fire-fighting doctors and the sick alike had only one hope: vivisection. Through the knowledge gained by it the conflagration could be doused. Through the medical advances it promised, those who had succumbed to illness were offered a life net. Antivivisectionist society women call out hypocritically from under bird-of-paradise bonnets for the 'life net' to be pulled away: a misplaced mercy for animals as practical mercilessness for humanity.

This striking image (Figure 0.1), which appeared in *Puck* magazine, a popular New York satirical weekly, captures what was at stake for medical science and society as a generation-long transnational controversy over vivisection reached its peak.[6] Its narrative, little studied compared with that of the history of antivivisection itself, was the product of a deliberate campaign, orchestrated from the heart of establishment medicine. The American Medical Association's (AMA's) Council for the Defense of Medical Research, formed in 1908, was to argue the case for animal experimentation in the court of public – not medical – opinion. The battlegrounds for medical research would be the pamphlet, the public lecture and the popular periodical press, especially targeted at women. In putting their plans into action, American society's leading medical scientists utilized the aggregate of more than three decades of experience, on two continents, to combat a determined opposition to the methods of medical research. This book is about that experience. At its core, it is about the strategies employed to try to cement an idea in the public consciousness: that the blood spilt in medical laboratories served a far-reaching human good.

---

[6] The image and its context are more fully discussed in Chapter 5.

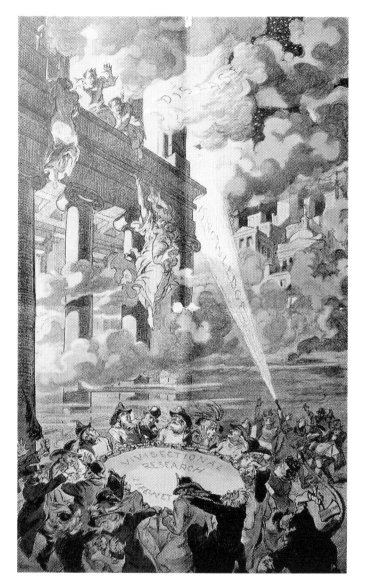

Figure 0.1 'Vivisectional Research', *Puck*, 1911.

There is no comprehensive work on the defence of medical experimentation that examines the entrance, in a coordinated and transnational fashion, of the modern medical establishment into the political arena and into the court of public opinion for the sake of self-preservation.

This is an astonishing lacuna in historical knowledge. Around the turn of the twentieth century, medical research was put on a propaganda footing, its power centralized in increasingly corporate non-governmental bodies. This is the essential dynamic that allows us to understand how medicine's experimental impetus survived largely unchecked, especially in the USA. The activism of this period set a standard for the way in which the world of medicine would talk to the lay public.

The story climaxes around the beginning of the First World War, but has its roots in the second scientific revolution, which was pregnant with possibilities for medical science, and in the processes of specialization. Physiology, toxicology, bacteriology, immunology and surgery went through great innovative changes, based on new experiments on animals, people and society.[7] The experimental impetus in medicine came from Germany and France. It gained traction in Britain around 1870 and soon afterwards in the USA. Throughout this period, beginning perhaps with François Magendie in France in the 1820s, medical experimentation was a challenge to morals, ethics and good taste.[8] We know remarkably little about how the medical response to such opposition was organized, implemented and networked across oceans and across countries. These are the formative moments in the development of modern medicine's public-relations machinery, which in turn reveal its political influence and social authority. The arguments of the medical establishment were complex, attuned to a particular understanding of experimental practice as an affective practice of humanity. Susan Lederer once wrote of American medical 'defenders of unrestricted animal experimentation' that they 'almost exclusively devoted their discussion to appeals to the clinical benefits accruing from vivisection'.[9] This is too narrow an interpretation. Medical scientists claimed an exclusive form of humanity in a carefully managed defensive strategy that was skilfully coordinated and built upon the lived experience of experimental beneficence.

Eminent individuals developed their defence of experimental medicine through a web of close-knit correspondence. Medical advances through vivisection, or the promise of such advances, had put the moral reputation of medicine itself in jeopardy. To combat accusations of cruelty and

---

[7] The classic reference is Geroge Weisz, *Divide and Conquer: A Comparative History of Medical Specialization* (Oxford: Oxford University Press, 2005).

[8] José Ramón Beromeu-Sánchez, 'Animal Experiments, Vital Forces and Courtrooms: Mateu Orfila, François Magendie and the Study of Poisons in Nineteenth-Century France', *Annals of Science*, 69 (2012): 1–26; Carin Berkowitz, 'Disputed Discovery: Vivisection and Experiment in the 19th Century', *Endeavour*, 30 (2006): 98–102.

[9] Susan Lederer, 'The Controversy over Animal Experimentation in America, 1880–1914', in *Vivisection in Historical Perspective*, ed. Nicolaas Rupke (London: Croom Helm, 1987), 241.

callousness, the medical profession set about publicly emphasizing its humanity. The modern medical scientist as far-sighted humanitarian was both a conscious construction of medical-establishment strategy and a deeply felt and daily practised dispositional attitude. With the formation of councils for the defence of medical research, the lines between propaganda and educational campaigns, between empty rhetoric and lived experience, were often blurred. Meanwhile, significant energy was applied to blocking the passage of laws that would regulate or limit the freedom of medical scientists to experiment as they saw fit.

In Britain, the USA and Germany, the medical profession did successfully control the public image of experimentation while simultaneously keeping legislation at arm's length. The book charts the specific ways in which this was carried out, homing in on the role of 'humanity' in successfully influencing both public policy and public opinion. It is much more difficult to assess the reception of this approach among the lay public, but there are key indicators of this at various points. Without getting ahead of the story too much in advance, it should suffice to say at this point that the particular construction and experience of humanity that medical scientists employed and advertised was often laced with a social, cultural and experiential authority that was further reinforced by allusion to exclusive expertise. Insofar as this is the story of the success of medical-scientific strategy in both politics and public life, it is also the story of the wielding of this authority: the cultural heft of a particular affect.

I approach this story in roughly chronological order, but shift focus to different national theatres throughout. We begin with the outbreak of controversy in England in the 1870s, before following that controversy first to Germany and then to the USA. We then return to England for the continuation of the account as it shifted ground at the beginning of the twentieth century, before resuming the story in America, where new strategies for defending medical experimentation emerged. Throughout, I attempt to keep the connections between the ideas and the personnel involved intact. While national conditions had a major bearing on the nature of the defence in each country, medical scientists and their allies represented, for all intents and purposes, a single community with a coherent moral economy.[10]

---

[10] Here I use the term 'moral economy' in the specific sense employed by Lorraine Daston, 'The Moral Economy of Science', *Osiris*, 2:10 (1995): 2–24: 'a web of affect-saturated values that stand and function in well-defined relationship to one another', deriving 'stability and integrity' from 'its ties to activities'. The moral economy combines *Denkkollektiv* and *Gefühlskollektiv*, which it expresses through social, bodily and professional practices (4–5). I have developed this approach empirically in *Science of Sympathy* and theoretically in *The History of Emotions* (Manchester: Manchester University Press, 2018), 190ff.

Magic

Medical-scientific research in the generation before the First World War modulated between the tropics of madness and magic, the monstrous and the heroic. Or at least, such was the range of its representation in public. For all their practical finesse, medical scientists grappled with the implications of both poles, and played a significant role in leading the public, and themselves, towards the magical and away from the mad.

Fast-forward to the 1920s, 1930s and 1940s and witness the high era of the doctor hero and of magical medicine.[11] In the preparation of this book, colleagues and peers frequently alerted me to this age of medical pre-eminence. The trope of the medical scientist hero in this period seems to be a matter of common knowledge. It is a matter of some wonder that, only a few years prior, so much seemed to be at stake, and a deep irony that the utilization of medical research in the twentieth century put such heroism in dubious ethical territory, justified more by nationalism and militarism than by humanity per se. But what had ushered in this apotheosis? Was it the First World War? Was it a particular scientific breakthrough that provided practical substantiation for biological magic? Perhaps both played a part, and I will spend some time working through the possibilities, but in general I take a more complex and *longue durée* approach.

The medical scientist as hero or magician had to be forged, which took time and fire. The process of fabrication is, of course, laden with double meaning. In this book I detail the ways in which scientists, through constant practice, constructed a new humanitarianism – a worldview that encompassed the elimination of suffering on a human scale – from the confines of the laboratory. The laboratory was a crucible of intellectual ideals, experimental means and emotional and moral ends. The results of this dynamic interaction were packaged and presented, in a circular fashion, as justification for the experimental method, and substantiation of a priori humanitarian claims. Experimental medicine – physiology, toxicology, bacteriology, immunology, neurology – aimed to salve and save, which in turn made the men who operationalized the experiments (their masculinity will be seen to be important) into saviours.

---

[11] For a general account, see D. Heyward Brock, 'The Doctor as Dramatic Hero', *Perspectives in Biology and Medicine*, 34 (1991): 279–95; Ross Mckibbin, 'Politics and the Medical Hero: A.J. Cronin's *The Citadel*', *English Historical Review*, 123 (2008): 651–78; Bert Hansen, 'Medical History for the Masses: How American Comic Books Celebrated Heroes of Medicine in the 1940s', *Bulleting of the History of Medicine*, 78 (2004): 148–91; Charles E. Rosenberg, 'Martin Arrowsmith: The Scientists as Hero', *American Quarterly*, 15 (1963): 447–58; Howard Gest, 'Dr. Martin Arrowsmith: Scientist and Medical Hero', *Perspectives in Biology and Medicine*, 35 (1991): 116–24.

It is important to state at the outset that medical scientists, by and large, internalized the humanitarian intent that their methods and materials signified, and believed themselves to be the saviours they claimed to be. A comparison of public statements with an abundance of private correspondence demonstrates a remarkable consistency. Antivivisectionists were denounced in private in less guarded fashion, perhaps, but the argument that antivivisectionists' humanity was false, while theirs was true, was retained. While this in itself is not a radical claim, it nonetheless needs to be stated explicitly because of the temptation to think of medical scientists as duplicitous, their humanitarianism a simple representational veneer that allowed them to experiment with impunity. I maintain that such duplicitousness, did it exist, would have resulted in catastrophe for medical science. Given the external pressure on experimental ethics and the scrutiny on the morals of experimenters themselves, anything but absolute conviction would surely have led to calamitous collapse. There were outliers: cases of ethical breaches and evidence of callousness, but their exceptionality was often employed to highlight the more general rule. It requires a complex analysis to reach an understanding of the making of and the feeling of humanitarianism in laboratory practice, or, put another way, of the lived experience of experimental sympathy and humanity.

Jutta Schickore affirms that 'Experimental reports are not a reliable source of information about what researchers really do in the laboratory', but helpfully the experimenters in this book left far more behind than their formal reports and publications about what they did in their respective laboratories.[12] They wrote, to each other, for popular publications and for speeches before lay audiences, about what they intended to do or had done, why they intended to do it or to have done it, how it would be or was in fact done, and what they felt about the whole thing. They rigorously scrutinized their own methods, as individuals and under institutional observation networks, and enquired into the methods of their peers, self-policing in private so that their public avowals of ethical high-mindedness would not merely ring true, but actually be true (at least as far as they were concerned). In this period, therefore, we probably know more about what researchers really did in the laboratory than at any period before this point. Moreover, we know how they felt about and how they wanted other people to feel about it. This dynamic, of the lived experience of the laboratory on the one hand, and of the expression of that experience, to different audiences, on the other, is critically

---

[12] Jutta Schickore, *About Method: Experimenters, Snake Venom, and the History of Writing Scientifically* (Chicago: University of Chicago Press, 2017), 5.

important. It provides for us the stakes of laboratory experience as well as an appreciation of the range of meanings and significance of the laboratory, as institutional medical science became more deeply entangled with public interest in experimental practice than perhaps it ever had been before.

The lived reality of experimental feelings notwithstanding, the other implication of forgery remains an important avenue of research. Much of this book concerns the conscious representation of medical science for a non-medical audience. This representation was, on both sides of the Atlantic, carefully controlled by medical scientists themselves and by close allies in the press and in high society. It was, in the face of stiff and often poisonous opposition, necessarily a highly selective and partial view of what experimental research looked and felt like. It dwelt almost entirely on medical success (to the point that experimental failure is subsumed under the narrative of a process that *always* ends well). I will argue that the aggregate of such material played an important role in feeding back on to medical scientists, lionizing them to themselves and bolstering convictions that were increasingly deeply felt. While medical scientists distinguished themselves by their access to specialist knowledge, specialist practices and a community of more or less like-minded experts, they presented themselves to the non-medical world of respected public opinion as pillars of progress, civilization and sensibility.

Here we encounter medical science as genre. Given this high public interest, much of the writing for a lay audience discussed in this book is not scientific writing per se, but writing about science, with the complicity and support of scientists, constructed often by lay writers for lay readers. It is not scientific reporting but scientific *reportage*, heavily editorialized, carefully packaged. This kind of medical writing about experiment is a kind of banal magical realism. What happened as a result of laboratory research, according to the standard plot devices of this literature, was nothing short of *miraculous*, yet miracles of this type could be thoroughly described and explained, if one only looked into the details (although the details were not typically supplied). The reader, therefore, was presented with a stimulus to awe, but commanded to ground it in reason, and to take such reason on trust. The humanitarian marvels of modern medicine were indeed the most modern of 'wonders': secular, worldly, technical, professional, procedural and empirical. To a large extent, they were also hidden from view, not necessarily because there was 'something to hide', but because of a lack of faith that the intelligent public was intelligent or experienced enough. When defending themselves before legislators, this defence was often offered.

Madness

Importantly, this genre, in its infancy, had to compete with its polar opposite, and was much less assured of the victory that would follow in the post-war years. I have previously written about the emergence of a popular discourse of scientific madness and excess that played on the heavy emphasis, coming from within science itself, on experiment in the mode of an unbounded curiosity.[13] The sequestered scientist, unchecked by social mores and lost to religion, was not likely to let 'I dare not' wait upon 'I would'. Poor cats. A host of other animals, including other humans, were the further literary victims of these men without feeling, these men of pure intellect and hardened hearts. From the early exemplar of Mary Shelley's *Frankenstein* through to the accounts of *Dr Jekyll and Mr Hyde*, *The Island of Doctor Moreau*, and the unfeeling scientist in *The Picture of Dorian Gray*, callousness and cruelty had become popular leitmotivs in literary representations of science by the beginning of the twentieth century.[14] The scientist monster in literature was drawn from anecdotal evidence in the real world of science, but also fed back into the real-world denunciation of scientists by their opponents, suggestive of a portent of moral and civilizational doom in their hands. Yet for all of these direct allusions to mad doctors and evil scientists, it was in another of H. G. Wells' novels that we encounter, by a sense of remove, what many believed to be at stake if the scientific vision be allowed to guide humanity.

The War of the Worlds was first published serially in *Pearson's Magazine* in 1897, being republished as a novel the following year. It was framed by the value of science and introduced in terms that would make sense to the popular scientific imagination. The Martians, with their superior intelligence, watched humanity with their own scientific gaze: 'as men busied themselves about their various concerns they were scrutinised and studied, perhaps as narrowly as a man with a microscope might scrutinise the transient creatures that swarm and multiply in a drop of water'. If men had an 'empire over matter', their complacency would be shattered by a species that claimed empire over them. Wells asked his readers, implicitly, to reflect on what they did, for 'across the gulf of space, minds that are to our minds as ours are to those of the beasts that perish, intellects vast and cool and unsympathetic, regarded this earth with envious eyes, and slowly and surely

---

[13] Boddice, *Science of Sympathy*, 58–62. See also Anne Stiles, *Popular Fiction and Brain Science in the Late Nineteenth Century* (Cambridge: Cambridge University Press, 2012).

[14] Mary Shelley, *Frankenstein; or, the Modern Prometheus* (London: Lackington, Hughes, Harding, Mavor, & Jones, 1818); Robert Louis Stevenson, *The Strange Case of Dr Jekyll and Mr Hyde* (London: Longmans, Green, 1886); H. G. Wells, *The Island of Doctor Moreau* (1896; London: Heinemann, 1921); Oscar Wilde, *The Picture of Dorian Gray* (1891; New York: Mondial, 2015).

drew their plans against us'.[15] This description, of the vast intellect housed in a merciless, unfeeling body, was a description commonly used against experimental scientists by their opponents. They sought, so it was claimed, a dominion over nature that went beyond God's will, usurping God, in fact, and claiming the earth for themselves against the better nature of compassionate, God-fearing people, who properly understood the duty of mercy and the quality of conscience. Wells captured a popular fear that experiment might extend to everyone; that rapacious curiosity would know no limits. This trope of a genius couched in madness was the cultural fabric into which antivivisectionist arguments were woven. To defend experimental medicine was to diminish these fears and emphasize, on the one hand, the miraculous ends of scientific work, and on the other, the greater good for which this work was done.

The Greatest Happiness for the Greatest Number?

What is the place of utilitarianism in this story? Much has been made, and rightly, of the greatest happiness for the greatest number argument within medical and scientific ethics. The utilitarian maxim drills down to the moral justification for experimentation, especially when experimentation seems to increase suffering in the moment. Experimenters forecasting a great benefit to humanity in the long run are not by any means limited to this period, nor did they invent it. But something is distinctly different about the ways in which medical science specialized and proliferated from the 1870s. The utilitarian maxim was, on occasion, doled out word for word. It was more or less always implicit. But most of the people who figure in this book did not self-identify as utilitarians *first*, and if we ignore what they said and thought about themselves in order to reduce them to a simple utilitarianism calculus then we shall miss the point and misrepresent what was at stake for them. Most, especially in the earlier period, rooted their ideas much more squarely in Darwinism (as it was, if this even needs to be said, not as it would become), and Darwin's contribution in *The Descent of Man* was a biocultural antidote to utilitarianism's cold calculations.[16] It implicated the human, at the level of feeling, of experience, as an emblem, as an exemplar and as a practitioner of evolved civilization. The moral calculus of experimental medicine was *lived*. As such, the claim that medical research and experimentation would have beneficent results in the long run was proffered as an article of individual

---

[15] H. G. Wells, *The War of the Worlds* (London: Heinemann, 1898), 1–2.

[16] Charles Darwin, *The Descent of Man and Selection in Relation to Sex* (London: John Murray, 1871).

and collective *faith*. It was a claim that ran to the heart of who medical scientists believed themselves to be, insofar as what they *did* was conflated with who they *were*. We could call this scientism and it would not be inaccurate. But the protagonists in this story would not (or not all) have seen it that way. Science was necessarily formational, through its practices, of a worldview. For all that their avowed objectivity has been demonstrated to have been an affect, this affect was nonetheless invisible to those who practised it.[17] The attachment of the medical scientists documented here to narratives of utility and to the rhetoric of compassion was no empty ruse. They genuinely believed, and their belief was built upon empirical grounds. It was a belief that could theoretically be proven by and through the laboratory. It was a belief that compassion inhered in medical research. Medical researchers were the vanguard of evolutionary development themselves, as representatives of humanity's most progressive state. Their influence, along Darwinian lines, would encompass the rest of (less-evolved) society such that society would enjoy the protection borne of the vision of those more advanced than the majority. It was the perfect entanglement of biological adaptation (in this case, mental evolution) and the power of cultural influence. Society was not in a state of nature, in Darwinian terms, but in a state of domestication, a 'garden' in T. H. Huxley's (1825–95) terms.[18] It was therefore subject to artificial selection, manipulation, an imposed set of constraints on future development. Medical researchers represented a major group of 'gardeners', doing what was best for society by virtue of their own evolved state, while limiting the forces of evolution for everyone else. The story of experiment in these years is the story of a lived experience and practice of bioculture. The blueprint was Darwin's *Descent*, as interpreted by an army of followers.

Importantly, then, this is not a story of civilization as defined by an ideology or a philosophy, but of a practice believed to have emerged directly from biology, into a cultural context that could subsequently be formed in its image. In her extensive intellectual history of utilitarianism Cathy Gere demonstrates that for this philosophy's protagonists, from Hobbes to Bentham, what lay at its core was an idea about human nature.[19] Government along utilitarian lines was about guiding and limiting that nature, to make the best of humans' desire for pleasure over and against their capacities to inflict pain in pursuit of it. But this view of human nature never had firm biological roots, however much the idea

---

[17] Lorraine Daston and Peter Galison, *Objectivity* (New York: Zone Books, 2007).

[18] T. H. Huxley, 'Evolution and Ethics: Prolegomena' (1894), in *Collected Essays* (London: Macmillan, 1895), IX, 1–45.

[19] Cathy Gere, *Pain, Pleasure, and the Greater Good: From the Panopticon to the Skinner Box and Beyond* (Chicago: University of Chicago Press, 2017).

depended on a biological foundation. Rather, biology was inferred from social and political behaviour, to which utilitarian ideas were a response. If there was a biological vision, it was of human nature in its most brutal form – rapacious, selfish, indulgent, *animal*. Darwinism reversed this. While Darwin undeniably tried to make biology cohere with social observation – it was made to *justify* the Victorian worldview – it nevertheless reached this point through natural history, seeing society as a product of evolution. And insofar as Darwin connected humans with animals in a chain of being, he nonetheless put certain humans (the most civilized of the bunch, like himself) in such a state of exception that the animal connection was distant.[20] If utilitarianism saw humans at their worst and tried to coerce them, Darwinism saw humans at their best and tried to let the best flourish for the sake of the rest. Gere ultimately underplays this. She notes, in passing, that Herbert Spencer ultimately came to reject utilitarianism's moral calculus, on the basis that outcome prediction was just too fraught in a complex society. One had, in the end, to rely on the cognitive and emotional *motivation* of individual actors – the best representatives of nature – whose evolutionary prowess would better ensure a good outcome than any kind of statistical or demographic forecast. Darwinism, which Gere largely overlooks, had, in the end, a biological explanation, and this explanation was at hand. Insofar as experimental medicine cohered around a moral economy based in turn on a scientific understanding of humanity, this understanding of humanity was expressed as a *natural* outcome of human evolution, limited to those men whose own intellectual adaptations had put them at the vanguard of civilizational change. Expressed this way, the rhetorical argument of the greatest happiness for the greatest number had even more power. For, it was not dismissible as mere rhetoric. It was embodied in these men who pursued it through their research. The condition of compassion, sympathy or humanity was the guarantor of a good outcome, even where in any specific case a good outcome could not be precisely forecast. This permitted the ambiguity or open-endedness of research, or of research for its own sake. Research, then, was not a utilitarian *argument*, but a mode of human being. As such, its practitioners embraced it as an undeniable force. It gave the strategic defence of medical experimentation a conviction beyond any paper philosophy. In fact, it gave it a conviction to match that of their opponents, whose compassion and moral conscience came from God. Here, then, is the most important dynamic of this story: two versions of ·

---

[20] Such humans represented an evolutionary saltation. See Boddice, *Science of Sympathy*, 163n14.

humanity, one naturally selected and enshrined in biological evolution, the other divinely designed and embodied, utterly undeniable to those who believed in it. In between them lay society, an amorphous and shifting thing, with its sympathies on both sides. It was here that the battle would be fought. It is almost a cliché to talk of warring for hearts and minds. In this case, both sides thought this was literally the case.

Experience, Experiment, Expertise

Humane Professions is about the strategy and tactics developed for an internationally networked defence of experimental medicine. In some respects, it is about the formation of a public-relations strategy by the medical establishment, but the analysis goes beyond the political and rhetorical to the experiential. Indeed, at the core of this book is the claim that the nature of the defence, as it evolved over forty years, was rooted in an entanglement of emotional, sensory, intellectual and practical involvement in the justifications for and methods of animal experimentation by individual members of the medical community. The defence was orchestrated to defend a meaningful way of life conceived on two different levels: the way of life of an increasingly professionalized body of medical-scientific researchers; and the way of life of a civilization that, in the view of the aforementioned professional body, was predicated on its activities. Humanity itself was perceived to be at stake in the defence of experimental medicine, and this meant that lived conceptual understandings of suffering, progress and humanitarian action were in play in rhetorical and political justifications for the continuation and development of this kind of research.

It is not a straightforward matter to say, in a pithy way, what the history of experience amounts to, but I offer this book as an exemplification of it. It draws upon the history of emotions and the history of the senses, but it goes beyond them, connecting them to the realm of ideas and reason, to practice (professional and bodily), perception, narrative and representation, to build an account of *meaningful purpose* and *meaningful behaviour*. Vivisection, to vivisectors, was practised in a meaningful way, with a positive moral valuation that aggregated the sensory, the emotional and the intellectual and, at the same time, amounted to more than this aggregation. The humanity that vivisectors professed, the encapsulation of their professional lives in narrations and representations designed for political and public ears, formed the primary justification and the organizing principle for the defence of those professions. It was a belief system, woven through a whole tapestry of subjectivity and collectivity that encompassed notions of moral fibre and character; professional conduct, status, theories and methods and the associated technical apparatus of those professions; class and gender chauvinism; work ethic; the veneration of an intellectual genealogy and a concept of eminence; a situated and specialized understanding of pain and suffering; an elevated estimation of the progress of civilization and scientists' place in it, leading it; and a dismissal of the beliefs of others (with a corresponding evaluation of the moral defects of such beliefs) where they failed to take into account the core principles of the production of knowledge, the necessary methods of this production, the clear humanitarian benefits of the application of such knowledge, and the incompatibility of such knowledge production with *sentimentality*.

There are probably many more things to add to this list of ingredients, but in enumerating even this much one sees the futility of reducing this account to a history of emotions or a history of senses, considered narrowly. The defence of experimental medicine was a way of formulating the experience of experimental medicine. It was a kind of incantation that drew from past experiences in the laboratory in order to represent its larger, humanitarian purpose. In turn, this fed back into the meaningfulness of continuing to design and perform experiments in the laboratory, where those representations were *lived* and re-lived. One might think of it as a compound of practice and preaching, of practical belief, of experiment experienced as humanity. The medical establishment talked so often, and over such a long period, about being humane because this state of being, in the terms in which they constructed and conceived it, prompted and animated their actions. Key to understanding the argument of this book is the interpretation of constructions of humanity not as mere representations, or rhetorical justifications, of vivisection, but as causes of vivisection and as experiences of vivisection. The medical scientists who appear in these pages experimented on animals not just in the name of humanity, and not simply to enact humanity, but as embodiments of humanity, experienced as a totality of emotional, sensory, intellectual, philosophical, professional and distinctly human meaningfulness. If we see the defence as less than this – if we see it as largely serving professional interests that covered over callousness, cruelty, monstrousness – then we misunderstand the level of conviction that experimenters brought with them to their work.

Humane Professions, therefore, goes beyond the creation of professional institutions of self-defence and beyond the history of networked collective action, to a situated history of the experience of being a medical scientist in this period. It takes medical scientists at their word, through a process of putting their words in context so that the meaning – their own perception of their own lived reality and its importance at a human level – becomes clear.

In unfolding the great lengths they went to in protecting their professional activities from outside interference, both legislative and cultural, we can see beyond a story of their professional self-interest to a story of professional subjectivity itself, and to the connection of professional subjects in a network of shared value and shared experience.

It perhaps requires me to say at this point that it is not for the historian to gainsay lived experience. When these men claimed to be practising humanitarians, it is not my place to say that they were otherwise, but it is my place to try to understand and demonstrate what it was they meant by 'humanitarian' in the context in which they employed the concept. I want to re-build this humanity from the inside, to see it from their point of view, and to see against what they were pitting it, and with what stakes. At root, *Humane Professions* is about the perception of an historical state of civilization, how to safeguard it and how to advance it. There was no consensus on such matters, but the medical establishment on two continents *knew* that the defence of experimental medicine was a key plank in safeguarding the future (just as their opponents *knew* the opposite).

There is another aspect to this focus on experience, which makes it a particularly germane approach in this case. For experimental scientists, 'experience' had become a central pillar in their capacity to know. Crucially, a lack of experience was equated not just with a lack of knowledge, but with an inability to know. Experimental research had made the biological sciences entirely *practical*. It was, so they claimed, only possible to judge the moral value of the knowledge produced from within the experience of producing it practically. One could not simply read about it.

This emphasis on practical knowledge, on experience as a means to knowing, was itself something of an ongoing revolution in the period here under study. If we examine, for example, T. H. Huxley's enormously successful text book for 'teachers and learners in boys' and girls' schools', the *Lessons in Elementary Physiology*, we can mark the changes, which are both epistemological and political. In the first edition, published in 1866, prior to the wave of antivivisectionist agitation that would arise in the 1870s, Huxley wrote in the preface that his 'object in writing ... had been to set down, in plain and concise language, that which any person who desires to become acquainted with the principles of Human Physiology may learn, with a fair prospect of having but little to unlearn as our knowledge widens'.[21] Reading, in 1866, offered a good chance of acquiring knowledge.

---

[21] T. H. Huxley, *Lessons in Elementary Physiology* (London: Macmillan, 1866), v.

By the time of the second edition, only two years later, Huxley felt compelled to add a new preface, containing the following qualifications:

It will be well for those who attempt to study Elementary Physiology, to bear in mind the important truth that the knowledge of science which is attainable by mere reading, though infinitely better than ignorance, is knowledge of a very different kind from that which arises from direct contact with fact; and that the worth of the pursuit of science as an intellectual discipline is almost lost by those who seek it only in books.

Of course, this meant urging those with a will to know into a practical course. Huxley's next paragraph would get him into serious trouble later, when the antivivisectionists would level the charge of the corruption of youth:

As the majority of the readers of these Lessons will assuredly have no opportunity of studying anatomy or physiology upon the human subject, these remarks may seem discouraging. But they are not so in reality. For the purpose of acquiring a practical, though elementary, acquaintance with physiological anatomy and histology, the organs and tissues of the commonest domestic animals afford ample materials.... Under these circumstances there really is no reason why the teaching of elementary physiology should not be made perfectly sound and thorough.[22]

By the sixth edition, in 1872, still prior to the outbreak of controversy, Huxley added another new preface, alerting readers to the addition of new images 'to aid those, who, in accordance with the recommendation contained in the Preface to the Second Edition, attempt to make their knowledge real, by acquiring some practical acquaintance with the facts of Anatomy and Physiology'.[23] In each edition, the previous preface was also retained, making it rather straightforward to mark the changes. Huxley would have to walk much of this back in a highly public manner, when accused of suggesting that the youth of the country should engage in vivisection, but the principle here espoused, that scientific knowledge was attainable only through practical experience, was retained and reinforced by the growing ranks of professional physiologists, toxicologists, bacteriologists and immunologists.[24]

This would become a double-edged sword in the defence of experimental medicine. One motive was to open the doors, to shine a light on experimental practices and allow the lay public to scrutinize what went on in the laboratories. The problem was that the aesthetics of the laboratory

[22] T. H. Huxley, *Lessons in Elementary Physiology*, 6th edn (London: Macmillan, 1872), vii–viii.

[23] Huxley, *Lessons*, 6th edn, v.

[24] For the controversy, and for Huxley's own problems with squaring the rational justification of vivisection with its direct experience, see Boddice, *Science of Sympathy*, 94–9.

worked overwhelmingly against the scientists. To allow the public to *see* did not allow them to *know*, but only to equate blood and cries with pain and pain with cruelty. One could hardly claim that experience was the only way to know and hope to demonstrate to those without experience that scientific practices were humane. This led to the opposite motive, to bar the doors and to tell the public and the politicians to mind their own business. If experience was the only means of acquiring knowledge, then on what basis could science defend itself to a public that claimed the right to hold science accountable for its practical ethics and for the moral qualities of its practitioners? Here, the scientists would revert to trust.

Trust us, they begged, for you, the public, know we are intelligent men, and our intelligence is being put to humanitarian ends. Some of those ends were repeatedly appealed to: the effect of animal experimentation on diphtheria, meningitis and other diseases; its positive effects on surgical techniques and on the elimination of post-surgical infection. The ends are good, they argued, so please trust that the means are good, and that the operators act with good intentions. Where understanding was impossible to share, trust in the humane professions of the men who did understand was, they argued, the only option.

This account necessarily conflates three closely related words and concepts: experience, expertise and experiment. To gain expertise one had to gain experience and experience, in this context, meant experimentation. It was a closed loop of knowledge production and practical activity. All three words share a linguistic root in the Latin: *ex-* (out of); *periri* (to go through). I introduce this book with the title 'experior' because it would have been a fitting slogan for the scientists here under study. Its five meanings capture the rationale of experimental medicine, its moral justification, its practical spirit, its intellectual exclusivity, and the principle of its defence: I test, or put to the test; I try, attempt or prove; I find out; I experience; I *do*.[25]

---

[25] 'Experior', https://en.wiktionary.org/wiki/experior, accessed 27 March 2020.

1   Darwin's Compromise

Darwin's Revision

Darwin published *The Descent of Man* in 1871. It contained the following seemingly common-sense sentence, so characteristic of Darwin's anecdotal style, his roundabout way of making his point:

> In the agony of death a dog has been known to caress his master, and every one has heard of the dog suffering under vivisection, who licked the hand of the operator; this man, unless he had a heart of stone, must have felt remorse to the last hour of his life.[1]

Had *everyone* really heard of this in 1871? Darwin gives no clue of the identity of this man, whether it were real or imagined, a trope of scientific cruelty that was somehow already in the air or a repetition of an anecdote on the lips of the chattering classes. As Darwin was writing, there were the first glimpses of antivivisectionist sentiment in public discourse, but nothing like an organized movement. This aside appeared in a long discussion on the evolution of sympathy, its limits and the possibilities for its extension. Darwin's sentimental note was published without an inkling that it might have political traction. Events soon overtook him.

By the time Darwin came to do the revisions for a second edition of *Descent*, the ethical landscape had changed. Darwin's common-sense aside had become politically sensitive. There was a risk, and not a small one, of it being used against him, to align him with his enemies and to alienate him from his friends and allies in the worlds of science and medicine. Darwin did not like pain, or cruelty or the idea that pain was intrinsic to scientific investigation, but Darwin did believe in the virtues of experiment, and he knew that physiology was at the centre of medical and scientific progress. It was the crucible of new knowledge about the human and other species, and it was the hope for new remedies against disease and suffering. He also knew,

[1] Charles Darwin, *Descent of Man* (1871), i, 39.

from his close friends and associates who involved themselves in experiments of this kind, that vivisection did not harden the heart or diminish sympathy. Given his position as the nation's, if not the world's, most famous man of science, of course he took the side of his friends and colleagues in the burgeoning controversy over vivisection. Instead of throwing away this line about the dog licking the hand, he amended it and, in so doing, captured the whole spirit of a debate that he would inspire and serve and that would outlive him by a generation:

In the agony of death a dog has been known to caress his master, and every one has heard of the dog suffering under vivisection, who licked the hand of the operator; this man, *unless the operation was fully justified by an increase of our knowledge,* or unless he had a heart of stone, must have felt remorse to the last hour of his life.[2]

It is not that Darwin, in between editions of *Descent*, changed his mind. On the contrary, Darwin's conviction about the virtues of experimental research were unwavering. It simply became necessary, between 1871 and 1874, to stress the point that the commission of suffering in the scientific laboratory could be justified, and without compunction, and without damage to the sensibilities of the scientist, on the basis that increases in knowledge were virtuous and necessary in their own right. What was not stated here, although Darwin made much of the point elsewhere, is that the vast majority of experiments using vivisection involved no suffering because of the availability of anaesthetics. Most dogs could not lick the hand of the vivisector because they were unconscious in the operation and destroyed thereafter. Darwin's point, then, was that *even* painful vivisection could be justified and, in the case of advances of knowledge, would be justified. What had happened in the intervening years that had required Darwin to make this amendment?

Born, or at Any Rate Bred, in a Handbook

The *Handbook for the Physiological Laboratory* was published in 1873. The antivivisection movement had been growing prior to this, especially via the pens of Richard Holt Hutton (1826–97), editor of the *Spectator*, and Frances Power Cobbe (1822–1904), who would become the de facto leader of the movement to abolish vivisection. But it was the publication of the *Handbook* that seemed to provide, to the opponents

---

[2] Charles Darwin, *The Descent of Man and Selection in Relation to Sex*, 2nd edn (London: John Murray, 1874), 70, emphasis added.

of physiology in particular, clear proof that the practice of vivisection had blunted the morals of its practitioners.[3] Its two volumes, the first descriptive, the second illustrative, were compendious in their descriptions of physiological experiments, compiled by the foremost physiological researchers in the country at the time. For all their thoroughness, they omitted any explicit reference to the need for humane treatment of animals and the general application of anaesthetics. To the almost immediate regret of most of the editors, these things were taken for granted. Moreover, they failed to address the context in which the handbook might be used, namely under the direction of men such as themselves in proper laboratory conditions. It was not meant for the curious youngster at home, but their failure to say so in the book itself was made to look as if the *Handbook* was a teach-yourself guide for amateurs, an outlet for the development of puerile creativity in the line of cruelty. The *Handbook* served as the announcement of physiology as an established field in England, immediately setting off multiple alarm bells. There were concerns about the Germanification of English science and, with it, the loss of English morals; worries about the calcification of public opinion, as defined by a 'new priesthood' of scientists; deeply held fears about the end of civilization, if tender mercies were abandoned to unbounded curiosities; and anxiety that cruelty to animals – for that is how vivisection was commonly represented – was the sign of all these things.[4] The charge of cruelty must be understood in context. It presupposed a motive of enjoyment or satisfaction in the causing of pain. The capacity of animals to experience pain played a large part in the controversy, but antivivisection can only really be understood if this question of intent is taken seriously. For, as the medical establishment would come to argue repeatedly, animals were put to pain in the service of humans in countless other capacities, from food to clothing to conveyance, and against these the antivivisectionists seemed not to cavil. It was, then, the practices of the *men* involved in vivisection that particularly cast a pall. The absences and omissions in the *Handbook* were seized upon as evidence of their societal danger, through their

[3] John Burdon Sanderson, ed., *Handbook for the Physiological Laboratory*, by E. Klein, John Burdon Sanderson, Michael Foster and Thomas Lauder Brunton, 2 vols (London: J & A Churchill, 1873). For the initial activities of antivivisectionists, see Rob Boddice, *The Science of Sympathy: Morality, Evolution and Victorian Civilization* (Urbana: University of Illinois Press, 2016), 54, 66, 73. See also Patrizia Guarnieri, 'Moritz Schiff'. On antivivisection and the *Handbook* in particular, see Richard D. French, *Antivivisection and Medical Science in Victorian Society* (Princeton, NJ: Princeton University Press, 1975), 47–50.

[4] The label 'priesthood' for scientists was in circulation by 1874, courtesy of Francis Galton, but was also used as a stick to beat them. See Ouida (Maria Louise Ramé), *The New Priesthood: A Protest against Vivisection* (1893), and Boddice, *Science of Sympathy*, 31.

callousness.[5] Still, a relatively simplistic formulation of animal cruelty was very often the rhetorical vehicle that carried these more nuanced and complex arguments. Much of the strategic defence of experimental medicine, therefore, would come to concern the removal of attention from the animal to the broader moral implications and societal benefits of experimental practices. Hence Darwin's revision. An increase in knowledge altered the moral weight of the vivisector's intentions. It removed the possibility of cruelty and replaced it with an implication of its opposite, for the accretion of knowledge in science and medicine was always, in the whole period under consideration here, connected to beneficent applications. Humans and animals alike could thank such an increase in knowledge for a reduction, writ large, of their suffering.

The heightened attention on the question of vivisection in England, and the spectre of its apparent rate of increase as a professional or, worse, amateur occupation, led to attempts at legislation.[6] Frances Power Cobbe was behind the drafting of the first Bill to be introduced into Parliament in early May 1875. It was not an abolitionist Bill, but it did propose to subject vivisection to the scrutiny of the Home Secretary and introduced the notion of licensing and penalties for failure to abide by the use of anaesthetics. In order to regain control, the scientific establishment drew up its own Bill. To defuse the antivivisectionist argument and to allow scientists to go on with their experiments, they suggested their own legislation. The intention was to regulate experimentation, not to stifle it; to give legislative force to the feelings of humanity that experimental scientists professed. In this act of compromise, of a particularly English form of incremental legislative reform, Charles Darwin was a major architect. In fact, the Bill was demonstrably subject to Darwin's imprimatur, though it quickly got out of control.

Darwin wrote to Huxley in January 1875, concerned about Cobbe's circulation of a memorial, for which she was gathering signatures, to petition the Royal Society for the Prevention of Cruelty to Animals (RSPCA) to formulate an antivivisectionist Bill. He was concerned at Parliament's 'thoroughly unscientific' nature and the likelihood that 'some stringent law' might be passed 'to check or quite stop the revival of Physiology in this country', which would be 'a great misfortune'. Still, Darwin was alarmed by the notion that anaesthetics were not always used when they could have been and that repetitions of experiments were made

[5] For the long history of callousness as a threat to civilization, and its connections to medicine in particular, see Rob Boddice, *A History of Feelings* (London: Reaktion, 2019), 131–63.

[6] The account by French, *Antivivisection*, 69ff., is still the best.

needlessly. If Cobbe and her allies were 'flagrantly unjust towards physiologists', it might still be in the hands of 'all biologists . . . to save suffering'. He suggested a petition, 'signed by eminent physiologists & biologists, praying for reasonable legislation on the subject' in order to 'counteract the passionate appeals of the promoters of the present movement'. He bade Huxley to canvass support among physiologists and warned that if 'nothing is done I look at the noble science of Physiology as doomed to death in this country'.[7] With this, Darwin assumed the role of defending vivisection, through the tactical method of legislatively regulating it.

Huxley agreed with Darwin 'about vivisection as a matter of right and justice in the first place, and secondly as the best method of taking the wind out of the enemy's sails' and set about engaging John Burdon Sanderson (1828–1905).[8] Burdon Sanderson then engaged John Simon (1816–1904), about whom we shall hear more; William Sharpey (1802–80); Robert Christison (1797–82); Henry Acland (1815–1900); George Rolleston (1829–81); William Gull (1816–90) and Michael Foster (1836–1907): the old guard, with the exception of Foster, who perhaps were most likely to share Darwin's mixed feelings of needing to defend medical science while at the same time being slightly cautious concerning physiology's experimental future.[9] A Bill was drafted by R. B. Litchfield (1832–1903), founder of the Working Men's College, who was the husband of Darwin's daughter Henrietta and adopted in Parliament, at the behest of Darwin and Burdon Sanderson, by Lyon Playfair (1818–98). There it would compete directly with Cobbe's rival Bill.

From the outset, Darwin's aim was clear. He personally sent the draft Bill to Playfair, who had already been given it by Burdon Sanderson, 'drawn up with the concurrence of some eminent physiologists' with the aim of serving 'to protect animals from needless suffering, & will not prevent the future progress of physiology'.[10] In this he was too sanguine. Playfair wanted a more 'humanitarian preamble' but told Darwin he had 'done a great service in the cause of humanity & Science'. Still, he had doubts about Darwin's attempt to safeguard experiments without anaesthetics by having each experiment registered. He thought it an 'impossibility' to 'explain to the unscientific the probable advantage of

[7] Darwin to Huxley, 14 January 1875, Darwin Correspondence Project, Letter no. 9817, www.darwinproject.ac.uk/letter/DCP-LETT-9817.xml, accessed 26 March 2020.
[8] Huxley to Darwin, 22 January 1875. *Life and Letters of Thomas Henry Huxley*, ed. L. Huxley (New York: D. Appleton, 1901), I, 470.
[9] French, *Antivivisection*, 71.
[10] Darwin to Playfair [before 29 April 1875], Darwin Correspondence Project, Letter no. 9909, www.darwinproject.ac.uk/letter/DCP-LETT-9909.xml, accessed 26 March 2020; Playfair to Darwin, 29 April 1875, Darwin Correspondence Project, Letter no. 9956, www.darwinproject.ac.uk/letter/DCP-LETT-9956.xml, accessed 26 March 2020.

any particular experiments'.[11] Here, Playfair hit on what would become a perennial problem. Scientists would ultimately get around it by claiming that such things were beyond the public's ken and that they should put their trust in the good character and moral fibre of scientific men. In the context of the perceived need for legislation of this kind, the argument seemed moot.

It was just as well that there was a short clock in the parliamentary session, since those practically impacted by Darwin's Bill started to see the cracks in it. As Playfair made amendments to the Bill, Huxley and others became aware that they might by accident outlaw all vivisection for the purpose of demonstration in the course of teaching, which would directly hinder them in their own work.[12] Men of science had risked legislating themselves into a corner. Burdon Sanderson, dismayed at the diversion of the Bill's language 'by men whose avowed object is the suppression of science' declared himself 'delighted' that 'compromise is at an end'.[13] Having co-sponsored the initiative with Darwin, he withdrew. Playfair was embittered by the affair, but in the meantime the government had decided to appoint a Royal Commission on the matter, and Playfair at least attempted to ensure that physiologists would be represented among the Commissioners.[14] The competing Bills were both dropped. Huxley received the news with resignation, telling Darwin that he had vowed never to 'be a member of another Commission if I could help it, but I suppose I shall have to serve on this'.[15] And serve he did.

It was Huxley who personally requested that Darwin give testimony to the Commission, for a man of such influence was a great asset for the cause of science. The Commission reported in 1876. In many respects, the entire story of *Humane Professions*, encompassing not only England but Germany and the USA, pivots on the testimony given to the Commissioners and on the actions taken as a result of its inquiry, specifically the Cruelty to

---

[11] Playfair to Darwin, 15 May 1875, Darwin Correspondence Project, Letter no. 9980, www.darwinproject.ac.uk/letter/DCP-LETT-9980.xml, accessed 26 March 2020.

[12] Playfair to Darwin, 26 May 1875, Darwin Correspondence Project, Letter no. 9994, www .darwinproject.ac.uk/letter/DCP-LETT-9994.xml, accessed 26 March 2020; Huxley to Darwin, 19 May 1875, Darwin Correspondence Project, Letter no. 9985, www .darwinproject.ac.uk/letter/DCP-LETT-9985.xml, accessed 26 March 2020; Sanderson to Darwin, 23 May 1875, Darwin Correspondence Project, Letter no. 9989A, www .darwinproject.ac.uk/letter/DCP-LETT-9989A.xml; accessed 26 March 2020.

[13] Sanderson to Darwin, 23 May 1875, Darwin Correspondence Project, Letter no. 9989A, www.darwinproject.ac.uk/letter/DCP-LETT-9989A.xml, accessed 26 March 2020.

[14] Playfair to Darwin, 27 May 1875, Darwin Correspondence Project, Letter no. 9996, www.darwinproject.ac.uk/letter/DCP-LETT-9996.xml, accessed 26 March 2020. UK Parliament, Report of the Royal Commission on the Practice of Subjecting Live Animals to Experiments for Scientific Purposes, C. 1297 (1876), hereafter, Royal Commission on Vivisection.

[15] Huxley to Darwin, 5 June 1875, *Life and Letters of Thomas Henry Huxley*, I, 471.

Animals Act of 1876.[16] This Act combined previous legislation on animal cruelty with new clauses that regulated animal experimentation for the purposes of medical or scientific research. It forced researchers to apply for licences and certificates from the government, effectively making the government the moral arbiter of questions of laboratory ethics.

I do not want to offer another lengthy account of the contents of the Royal Commission. Others have done so.[17] I will have cause to make reference to it in one special aspect, namely the construction of German monstrousness in the testimony, and the effect of this particular construction for German research (see the next chapter). To take the thing as a whole, however, the Royal Commission stands as the first ad hoc expression of the defence of medical experimentation by the medical and scientific establishment. As we have seen, there was a concern, especially among the older generation of scientists who were called upon to testify, that some regulative measure ought to be taken for the sake of safeguarding animals from pain. The overwhelming majority of practising physiologists and others who had recourse to animal experimentation testified that anaesthetics were already in widespread use and that vivisection had not dimmed or otherwise diminished the humanity of the men who did it.

The final report of the Commission endorsed this view, but antivivisectionists led by Cobbe harried the government for legislation and found, in Lord Carnarvon, an ancient of the animal welfare movement, a more than willing ally. A Bill was introduced that appalled the scientific community, which was rallied by Ernest Hart (1835–98) at the *British Medical Journal* (*BMJ*). In their supreme efforts to get the Bill amended, and amended with major concessions, they ended up providing tacit support for legislation that most had considered unnecessary after the Royal Commission. The Darwinian compromise had come to pass after all, but in an Act that was far more complex than had been anticipated in 1875.[18] Philip Pye-Smith (1839–1914) wrote in *Nature*, 'The evidence on which Legislation was recommended went beyond the facts, the Report went beyond the evidence, and the recommendations beyond the Report, the Bill actually introduced ... did not so much exceed as contradict the recommendations of the Royal Commissioners.'[19] It seemed, for science, a mess. The upshot was an awakening: the need for organization. Darwin's foot soldiers would

---

[16] 39 & 40 Vic, c. 77 (1876).

[17] Asha Hornsby, 'Unfeeling Brutes? The 1875 Royal Commission on Vivisection and the Science of Suffering', *Victorian Review*, 45 (2019): 97–115; French, *Antivivisection*, 79ff.

[18] The events surrounding the passage of the 1876 Bill are gloriously described by French, *Antivivisection*, chapter 5.

[19] The letter is signed P.H.P.S. so is presumably by Philip Henry Pye-Smith, the physiologist specializing in the skin. The quote, when it is used, is usually not attributed and generally incorrect. *Nature*, 20 July 1876, 248.

spend the rest of the century trying to undo the compromise Darwin had had a hand in making. Darwin, too, would ultimately come to see the Act as a step too far.

Monkey Business

Crowded into Gerald Yeo's (1845–1909) laboratory at King's College one autumn afternoon in 1881 was an astonishing collection of medical and scientific influence, eminence, intelligence and political weight. Jean-Martin Charcot (1825–93) rubbed shoulders with Michael Foster. Friedrich Goltz (1834–1902) was there, alongside his Scottish rival David Ferrier (1843–1928). Ferrier's mentor, William Rutherford (1839–99), turned up, as did John Burdon Sanderson and William Carpenter (1813–85). T. H. Huxley, seemingly omnipresent at this stage of his career, was there too. Here was a crowd known to each other, deeply embedded in each other's lives, careers and labours. They represented the zenith of scientific and medical expertise, covering ground from clinical psychiatry to neurology to physiology to evolutionary biology. They were there to see a score settled. Were brain functions localized? Ferrier thought so. He had said as much to the International Medical Congress (IMC) that morning, directly gainsaying the conclusions drawn from the vivisection of a dog by Goltz. The dog was also present at Yeo's laboratory, as were two macaques.

The monkeys, despite the illustrious gathering, were the focus of attention. Yeo had removed parts of their brain in order to demonstrate localized function, despite having started out a sceptic of Ferrier's ideas. Charcot was moved to remark that they were like his patients back at the Salpêtrière. The living proof being insufficient, the animals were killed and their brains dispatched to more medical-scientific luminaries, Klein, Langley, Schäfer and Gowers, for dissection and examination.[20] It was a career-defining moment for Ferrier and his science, but it was also the cause of personal trouble. The display, as well as the experiments that preceded it, became a flashpoint for the antivivisection movement and, in response, a motivating factor for the scientific and medical establishment in Britain to organize and institutionalize the defence of their methods, practices and rationale. Ferrier would be the first notable scientist to be prosecuted for cruelty to animals under the Act of Parliament that had been passed in 1876.[21] His

---

[20] An account of the debate, the excursion to Yeo's laboratory and the study of the killed animals' brains is contained in Sir William Mac Cormac, ed., *Transactions of the International Medical Congress Seventh Session* (London: J. W. Kolckmann, 1881), 218–43.

[21] There had been one prior trial, of Gustav Adolph Arbrath in 1876, but his prosecution was technical (advertising a public demonstration of the experiment, which in the end he

trial followed on the heels of a Congress that had been defined by a significant effort to promote the value of vivisection for humanity, and to do so in the name of a Darwinian vision of biology, evolution and civilization. Indeed, Darwin himself was implicated at every stage and had been something of a figurehead in the preceding years, as the medical establishment attempted to mollify opposition through consultation and regulation. While Ferrier's acquittal led, in turn, to fundamental changes in the establishment's procedures in heading off antivivisectionist and anti-scientific activism, this was an activism that had been forged by Darwin's foot soldiers and often in Darwin's name. This was a group of men, eminent in their own right, who understood that it was Darwin's fame and Darwin's principles upon which the general principles of scientific progress were predicated. The first decades of the organized response to antivivisection were framed in these terms, for the first time unfolding the motivations of the medical and scientific communities, not as Darwinists in the technical sense, but as followers and friends (largely) of Darwin who shared a vision of scientific practice that Darwin helped create.

In this, the role of the Physiological Society has been rather underestimated.[22] While its title seemed to link it to a particular specialism, such was the fluidity of scientific disciplinary boundaries (if such things even existed) that the members of the Physiological Society were made up of the great and good of biological and evolutionary science. Formed in March 1876 to protect the interests of physiologists, its first meeting at the home of John Burdon Sanderson included William Sharpey, T. H. Huxley (Darwin's 'Bulldog'), Michael Foster, George Henry Lewes (1817–78), Francis Galton (1822–1911) (Darwin's half cousin), John Marshall (1818–91), G. M. Humphry (1820–98), William Pavy (1829–1911), Thomas Lauder Brunton (1844–1916), David Ferrier, P. H. Pye-Smith, Walter Gaskell (1847–1914), J. G. McKendrick (1841–1926), Emanuel Klein (1844–1925), E. A. Schäfer (1850–1935), Francis Darwin (1848–1925) (Darwin's son), George John Romanes (1848–94) (Darwin's most ambitious disciple) and Gerald Yeo. The initial list of members was limited to forty men (later expanded to fifty) actively working as physiologists. The rules permitted up to five honorary members, and Charles Darwin himself was the first such. The society thus contained, from the first, Darwin, Darwin's family and his chief acolytes, as well as the majority of the most prominent medical researchers in the country. Obviously, with such ranks as

did not carry out) and did not resonate with the medical or scientific community. See French, *Antivivisection*, 201.

[22] French apparently did not consult Physiological Society records, concluding that in its early days 'the society qua society played little role in the activity' of combating antivivisection (*Antivivisection*, 196), breaking with silence as a policy only in 1881.

these, the medical community at large was within easy reach. In spring 1877, the Society started to investigate the working of the Act and found that certificates were being suspended and refused and that 'original scientific investigation' was being thwarted. A resolution was passed to submit a report of their investigation to the General Medical Council, apparently putting it in their hands.[23] But by the end of 1877, the Society was forming its own committee to report to the Home Secretary the 'effects of the impediments which have been thrown in the way of therapeutic experiment' by the Act.[24] Brunton was charged with rounding up the President of the College of Physicians and the President of the General Medical Council on the official business of the Society to personally remove from the Home Secretary 'any misapprehension concerning the suspension of certificates'.[25] By early 1878 the Society had resolved to 'take such measures, by issuing publications or otherwise, as they may think fit, to counteract the anti-vivisection agitation now being carried on throughout the country, and that they [the committee] be authorized to incur such expense as may be necessary'.[26] Direct access to the Home Secretary was immediately fruitful, with restrictions being lifted by such informal means.[27] The Society began procuring and distributing pamphlets by eminent physiologists on the subjects of their research.[28]

While the scale of all this was initially small, it was prototypical, and it was in the planning stages of the IMC that the Society began to assume a larger role, which in part explains the increased attention on animal experimentation that the IMC brought about. Romanes, Darwin's most faithful and enthusiastic disciple, was charged, as secretary of the Society, first to communicate with European and American physiologists and cordially welcome them to London for the IMC, and subsequently to invite forty foreign physiologists, ensuring the embodiment of a pan-European argument for the human value of vivisection. The Society was to provide hospitality and lodgings.[29] Romanes' letter (also signed by Gerald Yeo) expressed 'the hope

[23] Minutes of meeting on 10 May 1877, 31–2, Physiological Society Minute Book, 1876–92, SA/PHY/C/1/1, Wellcome Library, London.
[24] Minutes of meeting on 13 December 1877, 34, Physiological Society Minute Book, 1876–92, SA/PHY/C/1/1, Wellcome Library, London.
[25] Minutes of meeting on 13 December 1877, 36, Physiological Society Minute Book, 1876–92, SA/PHY/C/1/1, Wellcome Library, London.
[26] Minutes of meeting on 10 January 1878, 36–7, Physiological Society Minute Book, 1876–92, SA/PHY/C/1/1, Wellcome Library, London.
[27] Minutes of meeting on 14 February 1878, 38, Physiological Society Minute Book, 1876–92, SA/PHY/C/1/1, Wellcome Library, London.
[28] Minutes of meeting on 14 March 1878, 39, Physiological Society Minute Book, 1876–92, SA/PHY/C/1/1, Wellcome Library, London.
[29] Minutes of meeting on 14 October 1880, 56; 11 November 1880, 58; and 8 December 1880, 59, Physiological Society Minute Book, 1876–92, SA/PHY/C/1/1, Wellcome Library, London.

of our Society that the Congress of 1881 will intensify by social intercourse the friendly feeling which already exists between foreign and English physiologists'.[30] But the intent went beyond simple network building.[31] The presentation of a powerful consensus was in the offing.

As the IMC approached, the Society adjusted its approach. Romanes introduced Ernest Hart, editor of the *British Medical Journal*, to the committee meeting of July 1881. Hart, in conjunction with Romanes' nudging on the matter, was 'desirous of making some suggestion touching the policy of the Society with reference to the agitation on vivisection'.[32] He told them that physiologists had 'sufficiently long treated the accusations of the agitators with silence, and that it was now time to inform the public through the medium of the press what vivisection has done for physiology & medicine' as well as what it would do for the 'progress of these sciences'. The Committee, after a lengthy discussion, first set itself on a more vigorous publishing footing, proposing to republish articles on the subject and preparing extracts from the Royal Commission for publication in book form, but determined instead to wait and capitalize on the forthcoming IMC and consult with their 'foreign guests' on further action, keeping Hart in communication with the Committee.[33] The Physiological Society, in conjunction with the *BMJ*, essentially planned on instrumentalizing the IMC for the purposes of an organized defence of vivisection.

The consultation meeting took place on 5 August at St James' Hall, with the Society's Committee in full attendance, accompanied by an extraordinary array of twenty-two guests, including Goltz, Herbert Watney (1843–1932), Charles-Édouard Brown-Séquard (1817–94) and Henry P. Bowditch (1840–1911), who would come to play a major role in the defence of experimental medicine in the USA. At this meeting an international line of argument would be hashed out that would, essentially, outline the strategy against antivivisection wherever it might arise. The Physiological Society's resolution was read, to wit, 'that it would be desirable that a series of articles be published in a leading Review or magazine explaining the examples & evidences of the progress of knowledge by the aid of experimental physiology, & of the extent to which modern medicine

---

[30] Minutes of meeting on 9 December 1880, 60 and page facing 61, Physiological Society Minute Book, 1876–92, SA/PHY/C/1/1, Wellcome Library, London.

[31] I have written in great detail of Romanes' personal, private and professional activities as the early co-ordinator of the defence of vivisection in England. In lieu of repeating this detail here, see Rob Boddice, 'Vivisecting Major: A Victorian Gentleman Scientist Defends Animal Experimentation, 1876–1885', *Isis*, 102 (2011): 215–37.

[32] Minutes of meeting on 9 July 1881, 67. Physiological Society Minute Book, 1876–92, SA/PHY/C/1/1, Wellcome Library, London.

[33] Minutes of meeting on 9 July 1881, 68–9. Physiological Society Minute Book, 1876–92, SA/PHY/C/1/1, Wellcome Library, London.

is likely to be benefitted by physiological and pathological research'.[34] The *Nineteenth Century* was the Society's magazine of choice, and Romanes was instructed (through his own instigation) to contact such men as James Paget (1814–99), William Gull (1816–90), Charles Darwin, Thomas Huxley, Joseph Lister (1827–1912), among others, to write the articles.

Romanes sought out Darwin as a matter of priority, suggesting he write about the 'Mistaken humanity of the agitation: real humanity of vivisection', but badly misjudged the man. Darwin's support of the physiologists was unwavering, but he was constitutionally incapable of willingly entering personally into a controversy (again). He acknowledged that he had a 'duty' to express himself publicly on the matter, and wished for his name to 'appear with others in the same cause', but felt that he could not overcome his 'mental paralysis' to write anything 'careful and accurate' regarding physiology's achievements 'for man'. He begged Romanes to quote his letter to *The Times* in April that year, permitting Romanes to say that Darwin still abided 'most strongly in [his] expressed conviction' in favour of the physiologists. But he refused Romanes' request to 'stand among this noble army of martyrs' by writing anything new.[35]

Romanes turned instead to Richard Owen (1804–92), who complied, as did James Paget and Samuel Wilks (1824–1911). Under the editorial stewardship of Philip Pye-Smith, three articles appeared under the common title 'Vivisection: Its Pains and Its Uses'. Owen, though quite opposed to Darwinists in many respects, was animated by a concern about the status of scientists as respectable, honourable men. His essay dwelt on antivivisectionism's 'unproven and umerited stigma on scientific men', those 'choicest intellects' that 'add to the power of the beneficent healer, as applied to the prevention, alleviation, or removal of human suffering'.[36] Wilks and Paget, thus drawn into the controversy, would go on to play a major role in the defence of medical research. Other key figures in the Physiological Society would follow with their own, carefully placed, articles to inform the public of the humanitarian benefits of vivisection.[37] The IMC would prove to be the short fuse that helped formalize that defence.

[34] Minutes of meeting on 5 August 1881, 70–71. Physiological Society Minute Book, 1876–92, SA/PHY/C/1/1, Wellcome Library, London.

[35] Romanes to Darwin, 31 August 1881, *The Life and Letters of George John Romanes*, ed. E. Romanes, 2nd edn (London: Longmans, Green, 1896), 123. Darwin to Romanes, 2 September 1881, *Life and Letters of George John Romanes*, ed. E. Romanes, 124. 'Mr. Darwin on Vivisection', *The Times*, 18 April 1881 (and see below).

[36] James Paget, Richard Owen and Samuel Wilks, 'Vivisection: Its Pains and Its Uses', *Nineteenth Century*, 10 (1881): 934–5.

[37] Thomas Lauder Brunton, 'Vivisection and the Use of Remedies', *Nineteenth Century*, 11 (1882): 479–87; Gerald F. Yeo, 'The Practice of Vivisection in England', *Fortnightly Review*, 31:183 (1882): 352–68; William W. Gull, 'The Ethics of Vivisection', *Nineteenth Century*, 11:61 (1882): 456–67. Brunton, for example, concluded by stating that

To give a sense of scale of the IMC, examine the extraordinary composite photograph, produced in 1882 by Herbert R. Barraud, of the delegates (Figure 1.1). It includes 695 full-length portraits, for which there is also a key. The assemblage is a veritable who's who of the medical world in 1881. The keen eye will be able to pick out Lord Lister, T. H. Huxley, Rudolf Virchow (1821–1902), J-M. Charcot, Joseph Hooker (1817–1911), John Burdon Sanderson, William Jenner (1815–98), David Ferrier, William Osler (1849–1919), among the stars of the medical-scientific elite. The picture captures the gender and class dimension of the vivisection controversy quite neatly. Here are nearly 700 white men, ranging from the upper-middle-class professional and educated elite to the old guard of aristocratic and independent gentlemen of science. National origins seem of little consequence against this overwhelming homogeneity, which meant that science was implicitly being promoted as an act of male industry and effort. The appearance was given substance by the speeches made at the Congress, which supported or fed off contemporary evolutionary notions of men being the intellectual, active and creative sex of the human species, with emotions under the control of the will and the mind. They expressed an almost universal acclaim for the humanitarian benefits of animal experimentation (some of the distinctions in fine will be discussed below), which were opposed, at the IMC certainly, but more generally across two generations of public rhetoric on the matter, to the unrestrained emotionality and untrained, unschooled and undisciplined minds of women – even, and perhaps especially, those well-to-do women whose status afforded them the opportunity to speak what were assumed to be vapid minds.

The IMC, in the context of which the exhibition of Yeo's monkeys had come about, had, itself, been a signal moment for the medical and scientific communities in reaching a consensus about its position regarding vivisection.[38] A number of speakers took the opportunity to extol the humanity of experimental methods, which, coupled with the movement behind the scenes of Romanes and the Physiological Society, created an

---

'practically every important addition since 1864 to the remedies used to prolong human life and alleviate human suffering has been made by the help of experiments', continuing, 'it is surely not wonderful that we, who have the serious duty of meeting the demands of suffering humanity, should unanimously demand that competent men shall not be hindered in forwarding the progress of the healing art by one of its most indispensable means' (487).

[38] The coverage in the *British Medical Journal* captured many of the significant speeches. A complete record of attendees and their abstracts, with the exception of the physiological section, can be found in Mac Cormac, *International Medical Congress*. The physiological section was organized in such a way as to make it impossible to include abstracts in advance, focusing instead on discussion of 'important and general topics' to which papers could then be appended. Afternoon sessions were given over to demonstrations (vol. 1, 27).

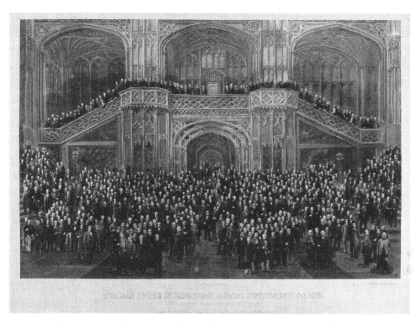

Figure 1.1 Members of the International Medical Congress, 1881. Composite photograph (1882). Wellcome Library, London. Attribution 4.0 International (CC BY 4.0).

impression of opinion in concert about the virtues of vivisection. I will have cause in the next chapter to come back to the speech of Rudolf Virchow at this event, but for now I will focus attention on a single speech, that of John Simon (1816–1904).

Simon is an important figure in this story. He was a pathologist, and conducted experiments on animals in that capacity, but by 1881 he had effectively taken charge of the government's public-health machinery. He had become the nation's first Chief Medical Officer in 1855, under the auspices of the General Board of Health, before a comparative boost in power, retaining his title as CMO in the Privy Council. He oversaw such things as the introduction of compulsory smallpox vaccination and had, as a professional role, the welfare of the whole population to consider. His organization of the institution of public health in a political capacity, as well as his endeavours to deliver public-health policies, are considered as major planks on the road to socialized medicine and, ultimately, to the formation of a national health service. His remit therefore also included medical research, and his name had come up fairly frequently during the first Royal Commission, to which he also gave evidence. In his capacity as CMO, he had funds of some £2000 annually to disperse on scientific investigations to better understand the causes of diseases in order to aid in their prevention. It was his job, as he saw it, to advise the public about the nature of diseases and how to avoid them. What he knew came from experimentation. So, while not all of this government money went on vivisection, Simon was still one of the nation's major funders, on behalf of the Crown, for those who wished to experiment on animals. John Burdon Sanderson was a chief beneficiary, and under him, Drs Klein, Creighton and Baxter. The relation to Klein, about whom more in the next chapter, would prove problematic, but when explicitly pressed on the question of the 'hardening effect' on character of performing animal experiments, Simon was confident that the men he funded were not adversely affected. He was asked, by Hutton, if the 'habit of regarding animals as a mere battery of vital forces on which particular results are to be studied, necessarily to a certain extent produces the effect of diminishing the sympathy with their sufferings', and answered firmly in the negative, noting that he did 'not anywhere know a kinder person than Dr. Sanderson'.[39] When the IMC came around, and Simon was given the role of opening the Section on Public Medicine, it was an ideal platform to make a broad case for the humanity of vivisection. He made that case with a lengthy lecture delivered with his colleagues in mind, but with the general public in view.[40]

Simon cautioned his audience that 'the general public overhears what we say' and, more generously than most of his colleagues, thought that 'the laity can follow equally with ourselves'. It was for the laity, therefore, that he set out his vision of the 'scientific method of State Medicine'. Even the concept of 'State Medicine' presupposed 'a special class of persons whom the unskilled general public can identify as presumably possessing the required knowledge' to inform the 'Body-Politic' that concerns itself 'with the health-interests of the people'. Its chief focus was on prevention of disease, and in the name of that cause Simon defended the right of the State to intervene and limit 'the freedom of persons and property' where the common health of the nation was at stake. In his view, 'disease can only be prevented by those who have knowledge of its *causes*', and there was no other method for the study of causes in the physical and biological sciences that 'that which consists in *experiment*'. Simon identified two options in this regard:

---

[39] Royal Commission on Vivisection (1876), 68–75.
[40] For more on Simon, see his *English Sanitary Institutions*, 2nd edn (London: John Murray, 1897). See also R. Lambert, *Sir John Simon, 1816–1904 and English Social Administration* (London: MacGibbon & Kee, 1963).

limited and controlled experiments on animals performed in the laboratory, and experiments 'which accident does for us' on humans and other
animals, without control, and with a heavy cost of human and animal
suffering. The former, which had progressed more 'in these twenty-five
years than in the twenty-five centuries which preceded them', were
offering 'larger and larger vistas of hope' through 'daily increments of
knowledge . . . a new world of strange knowledge'. Some of this 'abstract
scientific knowledge', he said, was already 'passing into preventive and
curative act', which was 'the same sort of boon' for mankind as Jenner's
employment of vaccination in combating smallpox. He did not stint on
praising the men, many of them in the room, who had made their age the
very pinnacle and promise of civilization:

I venture to say that in the records of human industry it would be impossible to
point to work of more promise to the world than these various contributions to the
knowledge of disease, and of its cure and prevention; and they are contributions
which from the nature of the case have come, and could only have come, from the
performance of experiments on living animals . . . at the cost of relatively insignifi-
cant quantities of brute suffering . . . to create an infinity of new resources of relief
for the sufferings both of brute and man.

Against this lay the Act of 1876, which 'virtually confounds together that
imaginary class of unqualified and cruel persons, and . . . our professional
class of *bonâ fide* scientific investigators'. In Simon's view, the names of these
men should have been 'sufficient security for their conduct', but instead
the minute scrutiny of the Secretary of State – a politician of no scientific
training – was 'substituted for the discretion and conscience of the scientific
investigator'. Simon could scarcely credit this lack of trust, in a profession
that had been regarded, 'from time immemorial', with 'the almost
unbounded trust' of the world. Simon forecast that the Act would have to
be altered and, in considering the moral aspect of vivisection, begged leave to
make a 'public confession of faith'. Examining his own conscience, he said
he did 'not in any degree regard it as a matter of indifference that, in certain
cases, by my own hand or by that of some one acting for me, I must inflict
death or pain on any living thing. I, on the contrary, think of it with true
compunction; but I think of it as good or bad according to the end which it
subserves'. Motive counted for everything:

Where I see my way to acquire, at that painful cost, the kind of exact knowledge
which, either in itself or in contribution to our common stock, will promote the
cure or prevention of disease in the race to which the animal belongs, or in the
animal kingdom generally, or (above all) in the race of man, I no more flinch from
what then seems to me a professional duty, though a painful one, than I would, in
the days before chloroform, have shrunk from the cries of a child whom I had to
cut for stone.

This broader, beneficent motive, this desire to save the many at the cost of a few, was too often overlooked, and Simon objected and protested against 'a standard of right and wrong being fixed for us on grounds which are merely sentimental'. He complained of the mobilization of 'an emotion' against vivisection that had nothing to do with what actually occurred in animal experimentation and took no stock of its motives. He felt that against such people, with such emotions, 'our profession cannot seriously argue. Our own verb of life', he said, 'is εργαζεσθαι [to work], not αισθανεσθαι [to feel]'. Here was the signal note, the defining motif of the medical establishment: a professionalized, restrained, diligent intelligence *applied* to medical problems in the name of relieving suffering, but, necessarily aloof from the aesthetics of suffering in the laboratory. What it *looked* like and *sounded* like was everything to the antivivisectionists, but nothing to such men as he addressed, who knew better. To them, to their 'standard of right and wrong', these 'lackadaisical aesthetics may seem but a feeble form of sensuality'. Against 'the mere screamers and agitation-mongers who, happy in their hysterics or their hire, go about day by day calumniating our profession' he harboured a bitter contempt. He expressed, against such people, a hope in education, and in the making of a population that would see State Medicine as representative of the 'true ideal of Government-action which sets its standard of success in the "greatest happiness of the greatest number"'.[41]

It was an extraordinary speech, coming from within the worlds of both medicine and politics, and aimed specifically to reach the ear of the discerning layman. The speech was published in full in the *BMJ*, capturing the tone of a medical profession increasingly alive to the challenge presented by antivivisectionists and of the necessity to strike an attitude and adopt practical measures to defend against them. If Simon tapped the spirit of the assembled company at the IMC, it fell to Romanes, in his final job with regard to IMC business, to prepare a resolution on vivisection, at the behest of the Physiological Section of the Congress, to be read before a general meeting at the close of the event. It was to give the IMC a post-facto purpose. The resolution, which encapsulated Simon's argument, read as follows: 'That this Congress records its conviction that experiments on living animals have proved of the utmost service to medicine in the past, and are indispensable to its future progress. That, accordingly, while strongly deprecating the infliction of unnecessary pain, it is of opinion, alike in the interests of man and of animals, that it is not desirable to restrict competent persons in the

---

[41] John Simon, 'An Address Delivered at the Opening of the Section of Public Medicine', *British Medical Journal*, 6 August 1881, 219–23.

performance of such experiments.'[42] With unanimous approval and a loud ovation, the resolution was passed. The world's medical establishment set out its stall in favour of vivisection as a humane practice.

Darwin's Regret?

The Association for the Advancement of Medicine by Research (AAMR) was established in 1882. The process of its establishment has been tacitly assumed to have been a coordinated and conscious strategic effort of the scientific and medical communities to structure its defence of medical research. Its activity is usually summarized as that of an advisory body, assisting the government with the adjudication of applications to conduct research by animal experimentation. In this way, the AAMR introduced a formal entanglement of loosely connected medical-scientific interests with government operations, acting as a private bulwark against an overly conservative interpretation of the 1876 Act of Parliament, and ensuring that the vast majority of planned research using animals was allowed to proceed.

There is something a bit too neat in this general reading, in part because it overlooks the way in which the AAMR came into existence. For this we must return to David Ferrier and the demonstration carried out in eminent company during the IMC. It was because of this that Ferrier would be singled out. Frances Power Cobbe's Victoria Street Society, the most strident of the antivivisectionist groups, had prosecuted Ferrier for cruelty to animals under the terms of the 1876 Act. The proceeding was a farce that ultimately damaged the credibility of the activists as well as strengthening the hand of the medical establishment.[43] Ferrier's debate with Goltz about the localization of functions in the brain had caused the delegation of men to take their leave from the IMC and head to Gerald Yeo's laboratory at King's College. It was Yeo who kept the two monkeys that had been operated on under his licence, and kept alive so as to test the relation of movement and sensation to parts of the surface of the brain. Based on a confused account of Ferrier's lecture and an assumption that it had been Ferrier who had carried out the experiments on the exhibited monkeys, as well as a further assumption that there was no licence to keep the animals alive after anaesthesia had worn off, Ferrier had been brought to book. The transcript of the trial, reproduced in the *BMJ*, shows that the prosecution was disorganized and

[42] *British Medical Journal*, 13 August 1881, 301. E. Romanes, ed., *The Life and Letters of George John Romanes*, 126.

[43] On Ferrier's trial, see French, *Antivivisection*, 200–203; Laura Otis, '"Howled out of the Country": Wilkie Collins and H.G. Wells Retry David Ferrier', in *Neurology and Literature, 1860–1920*, ed. Anne Stiles (Houndmills, UK: Palgrave, 2007); Cathy Gere, *Pain, Pleasure*, 150–60.

ill informed and the summons was quickly dismissed. No laws had been broken.[44]

As French details, prominent antivivisectionists such as Frances Power Cobbe saw Ferrier's acquittal as proof of the unworkability of the law, and set about an even more ardent campaign. But French is too generous in saying that Ferrier's trial was a 'potent publicity tool' for the antivivisectionists.[45] Whatever rhetoric Cobbe attached to the dismissal of the case, the evident truth was that the Victoria Street Society had misjudged their opportunity, overplayed their hand and been easily undone in the Bow Street Court. Although Cobbe protested that the Act was futile, it was actually an effect of the prosecution that would make it so. The attention it brought about caused the scientific community to reflect that generalized statements of the value of experimentation, such as Romanes' resolution at the IMC, were not sufficiently effective. A great outpouring of support had been occasioned by the public knowledge of Ferrier's prosecution, which began in November 1881, with a call for donations to support any financial burden that the trial might occasion. In the event, the British Medical Association met Ferrier's costs. The rapid dismissal of the case then led to further calls for donations for Ferrier, but with the intention shifted towards a testimonial.

It is important to set straight the chronology of what happened next, especially since French notes as *effects* of the Ferrier trial a call in the *Journal of Science* for a 'Biological Defence League' and the *Lancet*'s call for a concerted agitation among the medical and scientific establishment for public education on the humanity and beneficence of vivisection. While the *Journal of Science* did make such a call in December 1881, it was, at that point, a *renewal* of a call for such a 'League' that had been made as early as June 1880. On that occasion, the editors remarked upon the 'strange amount of apathy on the question'.[46] Similarly, the *Lancet* call for scientists to 'agitate! Agitate! Agitate!' was made in August 1881, after the IMC but before Ferrier's trial. So, who or what was the specific agent that broke the apathy and diverted the attention of the whole medical community towards the formation of a new association?

It was Samuel Wilks, the eminent physician, and one of Romanes' *Nineteenth Century* writers, who suggested (given that the Ferrier case was over) that the monies being collected for a testimonial to Ferrier would be

---

[44] 'The Charge against Professor Ferrier under the Vivisection Act: Dismissal of the Summons', *BMJ*, 19 November 1881, 836–42.

[45] French, *Antivivisection*, 202.

[46] French, *Antivivisection*, 203; M.D., 'The Protection of Research', *Journal of Science*, June 1880, 408; *Lancet*, 20 August 1881, 343–4; 'The Recent Vivisection Case', *Journal of Science*, December 1881, 733.

better applied to the formation of a 'Science Defence Association', to protect the whole community from such attacks from the antivivisectionists.[47] The renewed and ardent call for a 'Biological Defence League' followed, but it was Wilks' call that prompted action, and while French notes that the 'Physiological Society was clearly out of its depth in dealing with a challenge of this type', it was in fact the Physiological Society that facilitated the formal institutionalization of the defence of research among the scientific and medical communities at large. The Society, and Gerald Yeo in particular, was charged with administering the list of subscribers and monies donated. There is something rather fitting in this, given that Yeo's monkeys had occasioned the trouble in the first place. Thomas Lauder Brunton was instructed to write to Charles Darwin to ask him to become President of the new Association. Darwin declined on the basis of his health, partly, but offered a measure of support for the enterprise that was suggestive of regret. The tactics of the antivivisectionists in using the 1876 Act to bring a scientists to trial were seen as insidious. His attempt at legislative compromise, on reflection, had been a mistake. Such had been clear earlier in the year, when Darwin had expressed his views in *The Times*.

That piece – a reproduction of a letter addressed to Professor Holmgren of Uppsala giving his full opinion on 'the right of experimenting on living animals' – indicated that the whole saga of 1875–6 had been a mistake. Darwin confessed that he had been 'led to think that it might be advisable to have an Act of Parliament' to address the assertion 'that inhumanity was here practised and useless suffering caused to animals', to remove 'all just cause of complaint' while leaving 'physiologists free to pursue their researches'. Bitterly, he noted that the 1876 Act was 'very different' to the Bill he had had in mind. The Royal Commission, he said, had 'proved that the accusations made against our English physiologists were false', and he knew 'that physiology cannot possibly progress except by means of experiments on living animals'. Darwin expressed 'the deepest conviction that he who retards the progress of physiology commits a crime against mankind'. Perhaps, on reflection, Darwin felt he had played a part in such a 'crime'. Looking forward, he opined that 'no one, unless he is grossly ignorant of what science has done for mankind, can entertain any doubt of the incalculable benefits which will hereafter be derived from physiology, not only by man, but by the lower animals'. Darwin praised Virchow, as an example of a researcher who had saved 'many lives' and a 'fearful

---

[47] Samuel Wilks, 'A Science Defence Association', *BMJ*, 26 November 1881, 878. Some of the pieces of this empirical puzzle were facilitated by Kristin Halverson, 'Physiological Cruelty? Discussing and Developing Vivisection in Great Britain, 1875–1901', MA thesis, Södertörn University (2016), 59.

amount of suffering' and forecast that 'In the future every one will be astonished at the ingratitude shown, at least in England, to these benefactors of mankind'. Darwin committed himself to honour, always, 'every one who advances the noble science of physiology'.[48]

In that letter, however, Darwin had intimated that it was for physiologists alone to make specific claims about the humanitarian benefits of their research, concerning which Darwin was only an amateur. For this reason he had declined Romanes' invitation to write for the *Nineteenth Century*, instead referring Romanes to this letter. He now refused Lauder Brunton's invitation on the same grounds. He did not feel qualified to meet questions on medical topics, especially relating to physiological experiments, which he supported but did not carry out himself. It was not for him to be the figurehead of the movement. Around this time, Pye-Smith also tried again, and failed, to persuade Darwin to write a piece for the *Nineteenth Century*.[49] Darwin had already pledged twenty guineas to help Ferrier, but now offered £100 to become a life member of the new Association, suggesting that the President of the College of Physicians would be a better bet to lead it. This was in December 1881.[50] By April of the following year, this Association, now flying under the banner of the Association for the Advancement of Medicine by Research, had been founded and constituted. Following Darwin's suggestion, the Presidency was shared between the Presidents of the Royal College of Physicians and the Royal College of Surgeons. Darwin had died the day before the AAMR's first meeting and was celebrated in the minutes as a 'munificent subscriber to its funds'.[51] When the AAMR published its first list of subscribers in the *BMJ*, the late Darwin topped the list (not in terms of the amount given, but in terms of prestige). Darwin's £100 was topped by Bowman's £105, and matched by Sir William Gull and Sir Erasmus Wilson, while other luminaries such as Lister subscribed £50, William Jenner put in £52/10/0, the same amount as James Paget. These represent considerable investments and commitments, with the first fifty-two subscribers to the Association giving a total of £1138/3/0.[52] Subscriptions and donations continued to arrive, such that, despite a heavy expenditure on research, printing, letter campaigning and

---

[48] 'Mr. Darwin on Vivisection', *The Times*, 18 April 1881.

[49] Pye-Smith to Darwin, 19 December 1881, Darwin Correspondence Project, 'Letter no. 13566', www.darwinproject.ac.uk/letter/DCP-LETT-13566.xml, accessed 6 May 2020.

[50] Darwin to Lauder Brunton, 22 November 1881 and 17 December 1881, Francis Darwin and A. C. Seward, eds, *More Letters of Charles Darwin* (London: John Murray), ii, 439.

[51] AAMR Minute of 20 April 1882, Minutes of the Council and Executive, 4, MS.5310, Wellcome Library, London.

[52] *BMJ*, 1:1114 (6 May 1882): 679. Pye-Smith had invited Darwin to the meeting. Pye-Smith to Darwin, 18 March 1882, Darwin Correspondence Project, 'Letter no. 13729', www.darwinproject.ac.uk/letter/DCP-LETT-13729.xml, accessed 6 May 2020.

publishing, the Committee could actively invest £1000 by the beginning of January 1883.[53] The organized response to antivivisection was in far better financial shape than any of its opponents.

The direct line of events, from the over-zealous prosecution of Ferrier to the establishment of the AAMR, suggests that a major coordinated movement among the scientific and medical community had been occasioned by the antivivisectionists overplaying their hand. Their prosecution of Ferrier was miscalculated, based on a misunderstanding of scientific collaboration, the very meaning of the word 'experiment' (which was debated somewhat during the case), the operating terms of the Act, and the specific allowances of the licensing system. It did no substantial harm to any individual (though Ferrier himself was somewhat rattled by it), and in fact only strengthened both the cause and the fame of English medical research. Ferrier's victory over Goltz was something of a red-letter day. Yet ineffective as the prosecution was, it stirred the community to ask, in sympathy with Ferrier, what if this happened to another of us? It prompted them to organize on a much grander scale than the Physiological Society (though it could scarcely have come about without the existence of the Physiological Society) with the specific aim of protecting scientific research by means of experiment on animals in a whole range of scientific and medical disciplines. Moreover, it sought sympathetic and financial support from the professional community at large, whether or not they actively participated in animal experimentation, on the basis that medical and scientific knowledge, and the general state of humanity, depended upon this kind of work. Unwittingly, the antivivisectionists had sparked, for the first time, a concerted effort at large-scale organization for the defence of science, with sufficient force that individuals were willing to contribute to the funding of a new strategic organization.

The AAMR may have set out with education and public opinion in mind, but it very quickly became a shrewd, secretive and political pseudo-government agency. It rapidly went beyond an institutionalized lobby group, instead becoming intrinsically involved in the administration of the 1876 Act, to the great advantage of medical researchers. French argued as much in his 1975 book, but he had not seen the AAMR's own records, which are remarkable as a display of medical-scientific influence and authority. Despite the obvious conflict of interest, successive Home Secretaries signed over authority to a body of experts whose chief interest lay in administering the law with the least possible friction. As such, animal experimentation, curtailed for the five years after the Act, exploded in the

---

[53] AAMR Minute of 4 January 1883, Minutes of the Council and Executive, 22, MS.5310, Wellcome Library, London.

decades up to the First World War. Since French's account, which views both the Physiological Society and the AAMR through memoirs and Home Office records alone, and therefore obliquely, hardly anybody seems to have thought it necessary to appraise the narrative from the point of view of the medical establishment by actually consulting the records in question. The AAMR, for a well-funded and powerful organization of the medical community that actually administered the law, has received remarkably little attention since French, and then only to parrot what French originally wrote (whether he is cited or not).[54] While I do not intend any major revision of French's narrative, it does seem that we are missing an account of the AAMR from the inside.

The first Council and Executive Committee of the AAMR comprised nominees put forward respectively by the President of the Royal College of Physicians and by the President of the Royal College of Surgeons. Darwin's demise may have robbed the Association of a figurehead, but in his stead it could still boast the active participation of men like Huxley, Lister, Burdon Sanderson, William Jenner, Joseph Hooker and James Paget, who served as chair. It is an astonishing list, considering the influence it cast over evolutionists, botanists, surgeons, physicians, physiologists, neurologists and more.

Having formed, it immediately set about inquiries concerning the nature of its defence against antivivisection. The existing literature concerning the AAMR would suggest that it began as an organ for the influence of public opinion that gradually withdrew from public life as its influence at the level of

---

[54] The exception is Shira Dina Shmuely, 'The Bureaucracy of Empathy: Vivisection and the Question of Animal Pain in Britain, 1876–1912', PhD thesis, Massachusetts Institute of Technology (2017); for the rule, Nicolaas Rupke, 'Pro-vivisection in England in the Early 1880s: Arguments and Motives', in *Vivisection in Historical Perspective*, ed. Nicolaas Rupke (London: Croom Helm, 1987), 189–93, argues that the IMC was the origin of organized pro-vivisection, and while he references the AAMR records at the Wellcome, he does not extensively draw upon them, following French; Otis, 'Howled out of the Country', 42; Dan Lyons, 'Protecting Animals versus the Pursuit of Knowledge: The Evolution of the British Animal Research Policy Process', *Society & Animals*, 19 (2011): 359; E. M. Tansey, '"The Queen Has Been Dreadfully Shocked": Aspects of Teaching Experimental Physiology Using Animals in Britain, 1876–1986', *Advances in Physiology Education*, 19 (1998): 24; Susan Hamilton, 'Reading and the Popular Critique of Science in the Victorian Anti-Vivisection Press: Frances Power Cobbe's Writing for the Victoria Street Society', *Victorian Review*, 36 (2010): 77, 78n6; David A. H. Wilson, 'The Public Relations of Experimental Animal Psychology in Britain in the 1970s', *Contemporary British History*, 18 (2004): 29; E. M. Tansey, 'The Wellcome Physiological Research Laboratories 1894–1904: The Home Office, Pharmaceutical Firms, and Animal Experiments', *Medical History*, 33 (1989): 22n127; A. W. H. Bates, *Anti-Vivisection and the Profession of Medicine in Britain* (London: Palgrave, 2017), 135, reduces the AAMR to a passing mention while noting that the number of experiments carried out in Britain had soared in the period between 1876 and 1906. The oversight robs him of an explanation.

government grew stronger. This is not correct. Its founding *Memorandum*, published in 1882, indicates as much. The core of its argument lay in the following lines:

it is on the scientific investigator himself that the responsibility must ultimately rest of determining what is the best method of accomplishing a given scientific result, and by what means *the greatest possible result may be obtained at the least possible cost of suffering*. If restrictions are supposed to be necessary to control the conduct of careless individuals, let them be continued; but so long as scientific men exercise their responsibility in the humane spirit which has hitherto guided investigation in this country, they have a right to ask that no unnecessary obstacles should be placed in their way.

This amounted to demanding legislative change or at least access to the functioning of the Act, and the *Memorandum* did go on to express a hope that the views of the AAMR could be expressed in Parliament, in order both to rid the country of 'ill-advised attempts to totally abolish one of the most important methods of natural knowledge, and an indispensable method for the improvement of medicine' and to 'strengthen the hands of Government in administering the law, so as not to interfere with the just claims of science and with the paramount claims of human suffering'.[55] Such political intent was carried through in the AAMR's internal functioning.

At the first meeting of the Executive Committee, on 2 May 1882, two sub-committees were formed. The purpose of the first was to find the best 'mode' of promoting research, and it comprised Thomas Lauder Brunton, Michael Foster, Joseph Lister, Dr Payne, Pye-Smith, John Burdon Sanderson and Gerald Yeo. It was the most eminent circle of medical scientists. They specifically set out to find ways to promote research in physiology, pathology and therapeutics, agreeing that the chief way to do this was to 'remove existing *practical* difficulties', by which they referred to the problem of government licensing under the 1876 Act. To that end, they recommended that the Executive Committee should 'take cognizance of applications for licences and certificates ... and should accordingly put itself in communication with the persons authorized to sign certificates' and to ask such officials to join the committee of the AAMR. The sub-committee report was adopted by 24 May and a letter sent to the Home Secretary signed by William Jenner, James Paget and P. H. Pye-Smith. From the very first moment, therefore, the AAMR saw itself primarily as a political and administrative body, self-authorized to appropriate the practical operation of the law for the benefit of medical

[55] Association for the Advancement of Medicine by Research, *Memorandum of Facts and Considerations Relating to the Practice of Scientific Experiments on Living Animals, Commonly Called Vivisection* (1882), 14.

science. As an opening gambit, such a will to interfere in government business, concerning an Act that had been and which remained so politically charged, was audacious. Yet perhaps even the eminent sub-committee could not have imagined how well this approach would work for them.

A second sub-committee, with only three members and far less eminence, was charged with preparing lists of papers 'for reprinting and distribution', and this would be the visible sign of the AAMR in public life. Shortly afterwards, individual committee members were given specific roles concerning communication with the medical media: Brunton 'undertook the supervision and control of communications to be given to the *British Medical Journal*'; Gerald Yeo took on the same role with respect to the *Lancet*; and Pye-Smith the same for 'other medical papers'. The messaging was to be controlled, uniform and, for the first time, a representative voice of the whole medical-scientific community. Yeo himself went into print pseudonymously, publishing *Physiological Cruelty* in 1883 – a landmark text that defenders would draw on for years.[56] But the thrust, from the beginning, both in terms of investment of money and of minds, was to make the law work for science, behind the scenes. By 6 June, the AAMR had their reply from the Home Office.

The Home Secretary apparently jumped at the chance to avail himself of expert advice and assistance 'in administering the powers conferred upon him in the matter of the performing of experiments on living animals under the Act', soliciting AAMR views on the working of the Act and of the ways in which they would have it amended. After taking personal meetings, the form of this advice and assistance was to be stunning in its scope, a veritable coup for the scientists, and a hidden ace against all of the public antivivisectionist noise. The Home Secretary proposed that 'no application to him under the Act ... be entertained unless it has been recommended to him by the Council for the Association for the Advancement of Medicine Research'. In practical terms, this meant that all applications for licences to perform animal experiments were to be 'sent from the Home Office to you [Pye-Smith] at your private address ... with a view to their being laid by you before the Council'. By December 1882, therefore, the AAMR had become a de facto agent of the government, in charge of both fielding and recommending licence applications, with the Home Office transforming its own

---

[56] Philanthropos [Gerald Yeo], *Physiological Cruelty; or, Fact v. Fancy: An Inquiry into the Vivisection Question* (London: Tinsley, 1883). Yeo offered 300 copies of 'his book' to the AAMR in lieu of paying his subscription that year. AAMR Minute book, 45. Romanes was one of its most praiseworthy reviewers, lauding its author as 'something more (and may we not say something better?) than a man of science and a logician. He is clearly a man of large and generous heart, of finely strung feelings, and a lover of animals as well as a "lover of men"'. George John Romanes, 'Physiological Cruelty', *Nature*, 28 (1883): 537–8.

role from that of official adjudicator on experimental science to that of rubber stamp.

The arrangement, which had been properly fleshed out by January 1883, did not prevent the AAMR from promoting experimental medicine in other ways and nor did it oblige AAMR members to recuse themselves from recommending the granting of licences for which they were the applicants. Indeed, the AAMR's stated role was to make 'practical suggestions' on applications for the sake of removing delays in the system. Applications could arise from within the AAMR membership, be passed to the AAMR for expert approval or revision before approval, and then sent back to the Home Office for granting. For example, an early application under this scheme came from Heneage Gibbes, who had studied under Emanuel Klein, but the co-signers of the application were John Burdon Sanderson and William Jenner, both members of the Executive Committee that then recommended the granting of the licence.[57] Correspondence would be filtered through a formal address at the Royal College of Physicians, and applications managed by a permanent sub-committee and a secretary on 100 Guineas a year. In cases where there might have been doubts, the AAMR resolved not to pass applications back to the Home Office until any necessary revisions had been carried out. They therefore practically eliminated any chance of applications being refused.[58] For example, one report in support of an application for experiments on dogs was sent by the Home Office to a government appointed inspector, who in turn reported that he was 'unable to see any reason for believing that the experiments proposed ... are calculated, so far as they have any worth, to advance knowledge either practically or scientifically' and that the experiments 'would be attended with considerable suffering, in all probability greater than would be commensurate with any utility to be derived from them'. With such stark condemnation, the Home Office simply asked the AAMR for 'further observations' and the Committee quickly resolved that the application 'be supported'.[59] A letter quickly followed, 'stating at full length

---

[57] AAMR Minute of 27 February 1883, Minutes of the Council and Executive, 27, MS.5310, Wellcome Library, London.

[58] AAMR Minute of 27 February 1883, Minutes of the Council and Executive, 28, MS.5310, Wellcome Library, London. There was the occasional wrinkle, as with the applications of Yeo and Lockhart Gibson, which had been refused despite significant pressure from the AAMR. They had applied for certificate E, which was specifically for experiments involving cats and dogs without the use of anaesthesia, the most politically and ethically challenging of all categories of research licensing under the Act. AAMR Minutes of 11 January and 15 February 1884, Minutes of the Council and Executive, 32–3, MS.5310, Wellcome Library, London. For how this specific argument with the Home Office played out, see Shmuely, 'Bureaucracy of Empathy', 96–100.

[59] AAMR Minute of 2 February 1886, Minutes of the Council and Executive, 40, MS.5310, Wellcome Library, London.

the arguments in favour of it and the grounds in which it received the support of the Association'. Within a week, the Home Secretary had granted the licence and certificate B. Lay opinion about suffering, about utility and about the value of experiments for the production of knowledge, could thus be simply swept away by the authority of expertise, delivered in concert through its institutionalization in the AAMR.[60]

There was a massive conflict of interest. The relationship was not publicly acknowledged (indeed, communication from the Home Office was marked 'Pressing & Confidential'), but it was congenial. At one point in the middle of 1883, the sub-committee charged with dealing with applications and communication with the Home Office reported that 'relations of the Assoc. with the H.O. were at the present time in every way satisfactory and that all communications from the Assoc. received marked courtesy and attention. In one instance, an answer to a pressing request the Home Secretary granted a license and allowed a Certificate B in 2 days'.[61] Medical science had, almost by the power of its own authority with Parliament, safeguarded the growth of experimental medicine irrespective of the restrictive Act by becoming custodian of that Act.

This is all remarkable in its own right, but the AAMR's quickly discovered power should cause a re-assessment of the standard rhetorical lines of argument of the medical-scientific community from 1882 down the First World War. After 1876, it had quickly become orthodox to proclaim in public that the Act had shackled and frustrated medical science, to the great detriment of the pursuit of knowledge and the public good. That had been the leitmotiv of the IMC in 1881, and it coloured the public animadversions of medical scientists for a generation. But behind the scenes, the AAMR had effectively removed any barrier to the continuation and development of experimental research. Complaining about the Act became a device to make sure that no further inroads into experimental freedom could be made by antivivisectionists. If 1876 could be represented as a terrible burden, then it could be used to blunt more radical antivivisectionist cant. The public could be reassured that the antivivisectionists had already won their great victory. In fact, the 1876 Act was a dead letter.

This reappraisal must also throw the other activities of the AAMR and its successor, the Research Defence Society (see Chapter 4) into new light. For while it remains fair to say that the members of the AAMR did consider antivivisectionism a real threat, the arrangement with the Home Office

[60] AAMR Minute of 21 May 1886, Minutes of the Council and Executive, 41, MS.5310, Wellcome Library, London.
[61] AAMR Minute of 25 June 1883, Minutes of the Council and Executive, 30–31, MS.5310, Wellcome Library, London.

allowed them to promote research in other ways with even more power. For example, in the same sub-committee report that advised the AAMR to seek the ear of the Home Secretary, it was also advised that research be directly funded from AAMR coffers, perhaps even to the extent of sponsoring a laboratory in the field of therapeutics, and with specific intentions to fund research on the causes of tuberculosis. In their second meeting, the sub-committee resolved to request £300 to cover the personal remuneration of an investigator, over the course of three years, plus expenses, to carry out this work. In addition, they suggested a grant of £100 to Scottish bacteriologist William Watson Cheyne (1852–1932) to pursue the work of Robert Koch (1843–1910) and Jean Joseph Henri Toussaint (1847–90) on the subject. This included funding for departure from England to follow up directly with Koch. Cheyne's work, once vetted, was then slated for publication in the *Practitioner*, with additional funds from the Association to copy and distribute it, with interest generated by the posting of an abstract of the research in the prominent medical weeklies.[62]

A further recommendation was made to grant financial support to Charles S. Roy (1854–97) for his research on foot and mouth disease. A close examination of AAMR records shows that the funding of research in this case was directly politically motivated, as a response to Roy's vilification by antivivisectionists towards the end of 1882. Roy himself had been introduced to a meeting of the Executive Committee, laying upon the table a series of pamphlets and articles, among them a prominent piece by Frances Power Cobbe in the *Contemporary Review*, that served to highlight the cruelty of Roy's experiments on the innervation of the kidney, which he had described to the IMC in 1881. There was also an anonymously published piece that called his character into question. The Committee prepared and issued a statement vindicating Roy, for which Roy expressed his gratitude. If this were as far the AAMR had gone in such matters, then it might simply have become a pressure group, seeking to influence public opinion in the exact same manner as the antivivisection societies. But in its capacity also to fund research, the AAMR could add material weight to its defence of researchers' characters, by directly funding their research and by ensuring that there would be no barriers to the securing of licences. Roy received £200 from Association funds.[63] He would be funded again in 1885, to investigate the Spanish cholera outbreak.[64]

---

[62] AAMR Minute of 27 February 1883, Minutes of the Council and Executive, 27, MS.5310, Wellcome Library, London.

[63] AAMR Minute of 11 January 1884, Minutes of the Council and Executive, 32, MS.5310, Wellcome Library, London.

[64] French, *Antivivisection*, 205–6; AAMR Minute of 28 September 1885, Minutes of the Council and Executive, 38, MS.5310, Wellcome Library, London.

At Executive Committee meetings it was not uncommon for sitting MPs to be present, by invitation, and for discussions to take place as to the best ways to thwart any new attempts at antivivisectionist legislation. In 1883, for example, R. T. Reid (1846–1923) put forward a Bill for the abolition of vivisection (it was not his first attempt and would not be his last). It never stood a chance of success, given government opposition, but it still afforded an opportunity for the AAMR to exert its influence on public opinion. The Presidents of the Royal Colleges of Physicians and Surgeons could be prevailed upon, for example, to publish letters of opposition in *The Times*, directed through the discussions of the Committee.[65] Sir Lyon Playfair's speech in the House of Commons was, with his permission, printed and distributed not only to AAMR members, but to all members of the legislature.[66] This snapshot of the AAMR's behind-the-scenes activity shows it to have been a slick operation that was defined by conflict of interest, defending character in public, funding research in private, and facilitating research by acting as an arm of government, in a semi-official capacity. All the while, the AAMR devoted considerable time and money to the publication or re-publication and distribution of literature dedicated to the cause of promoting experimental science and medicine using live animals.

While French has characterized an apparent diminution of such sponsored literature by the end of the 1880s as indicative of the AAMR's assumed role of administrator of the 1876 Act, it is more likely that there was simply less need for such literature by the beginning of the 1890s, and fewer funds to pursue such a course. 1881 had proven to be a great flashpoint in the controversy, but the antivivisectionist cause had been thwarted in court, and then utterly out-manoeuvred by the medical establishment. While the beginning of the twentieth century would see renewed ardour among the antivivisectionists, as well as some long-overdue scrutiny of AAMR ethics, and while individual scientists occasionally ran into administrative difficulties with the working of the Act, it seems reasonable to conclude that the AAMR had effectively ushered in a period of great expansion of experimental work, with little recourse for its opponents in return. Darwin's foot soldiers, helped in no small degree by Darwin's financial legacy, had won a major temporary victory in the defence of experimental medicine.

Nevertheless, the considerable expenditure on research grants, printing and publishing had, despite the AAMR's obvious success among the

---

[65] AAMR Minute of 2 April 1883, Minutes of the Council and Executive, 29, MS.5310, Wellcome Library, London. William Jenner and T. Spencer Wells, 'The Abolition of Vivisection', *The Times*, 3 April 1883.

[66] AAMR Minute of 25 June 1883, Minutes of the Council and Executive, 30, MS.5310, Wellcome Library, London.

medical community, put the Association in financial difficulties by the beginning of 1888. It boasted only about £100 in funds and thereafter it offered much less support to active researchers, focusing its efforts on the support of applications for licences and certificates for research from the Home Office. Contra French's interpretation, that the AAMR retreated into silence as a deliberate strategy, it seems more likely that it simply found it impossible to continue its breadth of activities after the initial influx of cash had been dispensed. What the Committee retained was a significant expertise and influence, which it could bring to bear on the Home Office on behalf of scientists active in the field. This came with minimal cost. At the end of 1889 the Association declared itself unable to make any grants, and in 1891, Stephen Paget (1855–1926), the Association Secretary and the son of James, requested that his own salary not exceed £50.[67] It was becoming a tight ship, but the principal usefulness of the Association still lay in its capacity to influence the Home Secretary, up to the point of changing his mind about proposals for experiments that were initially refused. But basic subscriptions barely covered costs, and there were no more large capital donations, like Darwin's, that had launched the Association with such fanfare. In part, this was a result of the Association's clear success. It had made experimental research possible in Britain, to an extent scarcely imaginable in 1876, or even in 1881. It had done so while depending entirely upon the scientific and medical community, and had limited itself to communicating only with that body of professionals. As the scene shifted again, in the early twentieth century, the defence of experiment would have to look, for the first time in a substantial way, beyond the professional community to the lay public. Here, it would find new strategies and new modes of defence, and, importantly, new revenue streams, while reproducing old rhetorical scripts.

[67] AAMR Minute of 8 November 1889 and Minute of 18 June 1891, Minutes of the Council and Executive, 61, 66, MS.5310, Wellcome Library, London.

2   Medical Monsters?

Sentimentality, Head and Heart

The Czech-born, Austrian painter Gabriel von Max (1840–1915) captured, in 1883, the affective argument that was being spun around the contested practice of vivisection in the German-speaking lands of continental Europe. Figure 2.1, *Der Vivisector* (The Vivisector), here in a photogravure of 1886, after an etching of Max's original by M. J. Holzapfl, shows the characteristically bearded and bespectacled physiologist, scalpel still in hand, caught by surprise by the embodiment of Compassion. The object of research, a small dog, still muzzled with cord, has been snatched into the right arm of Compassion, who holds aloft in the other hand the scales of justice. In those scales sit, on one side, a laureled brain, signifying glorious knowledge; on the other side sits the burning heart, seat of love and compassion. Tellingly, the heart weighs heavier in the balance. The physiologist, thus judged, is found to have sacrificed his tender mercies for the sake of knowledge without wisdom. His curiosity has resulted in callousness. The implication is simple enough: one cannot leave scientists to make humane or compassionate decisions. Such decisions must be made for them. Compassion, from without, must intervene.

While I will not dwell at any length on antivivisectionist arguments, this image is particularly striking for its engagement with and gainsaying of scientific arguments about the humanity of medical research. Indeed, there are many instances of images like this, especially in England and the USA, where exactly the reverse argument is presented. True humanity is embodied in the production of knowledge, which surpasses the heart in its ability to practice compassion. The context of such depictions tend to withdraw from an acute focus on physiologist and animal subject to the general state of suffering humanity and the prospects for its succour. Max's image, by such reasoning, perfectly encapsulates what the medical scientists would

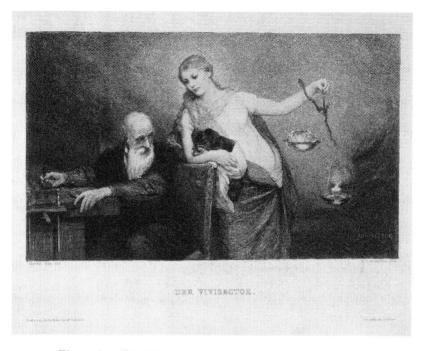

Figure 2.1 'Der Vivisector', Gabriel Max, 1886. Wellcome Library, London. Attribution 4.0 International (CC BY 4.0).

call the 'false humanity' or 'sentimentality' of the antivivisection move-ment. When the painting was exhibited in London in 1885, it was given the title 'The Genius of Pity staying the Vivisector's hand'. The argu-ment had international resonance then, but scientists would mock and diminish such references to pity as self-indulgent luxuriating.[1] It focused the sentimental on her own heart or conscience and made her – almost always *her* – unable to see the true causes or extent of suffering, and the most likely source of its remedy.

[1] Alexander Bain, *Emotions and the Will*, 3rd edn (London: Longmans, Green, 1875), 142–44, understood the 'luxury of pity' as self-indulgent compassion, but nonetheless ordinarily necessary. Herbert Spencer picked up on Bain's phrase and denounced it as a root of sentimentality and of what he called 'ego-altruism', a feeling excited by 'some-thing feeble and dependent to be taken care of', like the little girl 'with her doll', or the 'lady with her lap-dog'. It was, while 'natural', *pathetic*. All of this would be undone by new knowledge about the evolution of moral sentiments and of the evolution of moral senti-ments themselves. The scientist was, literally, superior to this so-called genius of pity. See Herbert Spencer, *Principles of Psychology* (1899; Osnabrück: Otto Zeller, 1966), ii, 688–92.

If the narrative of Max's painting was in the ascendency in 1883, by the turn of the century the argument of the medical scientists was equally prevalent, if not more so, and their argument was holding sway. As evidence, by way of a pictorial framing that darkly mirrors the painting of Max, take this image that appeared in the satirical German magazine *Lustiger Blätter* in 1899 (Figure 2.2).[2] It not only fully understands the argument of the scientists, but assumes that the argument is well enough known by the general public for it to be successfully inverted in a humorous manner. The image shows a physiological teaching theatre, but the students and experimenters are all animals normally found strapped to the cutting boards: rabbits, dogs, rats, frogs and so on. On the board, the experimental animal is a bound human, bearded and bespectacled, per the physiologist trope, but actually looking strikingly like Robert Koch, who would have been known broadly. Koch's fame was long-standing, especially in the world of epidemiology, public health, microbiology and bacteriology. He would win the Nobel Prize in 1905, and was, when this picture was published, the Director of the Preußisches Institut für Infektionskrankheiten, which had been founded for the purpose of housing Koch's research. Paul Ehrlich (1854–1915), who is also a candidate for the man on the vivisection table, worked there under Koch.

The caption for this satirical cartoon is an excellent satire: 'The Vivisection of Humans: Professor Kanickulus: Only no false sentimentality! The principle of the freedom of research demands that I vivisect this human for the health of the whole world of animals!' It understands that the question of humanity was at stake in this debate, and it gently mocks the antivivisectionists through a quite ridiculous reversal. While the image can hardly be said to be supportive of medical experimentation on animals, it nevertheless foregrounds the question of where proper sentiment should lie, for few readers would have sympathized with the idea of sacrificing a man for the sake of animal health, but most would have been on board with the idea of the opposite.

The two images show the rhetorical (and pictorial) field of arguments about vivisection. They did not hinge on what, specifically, was done or found in the laboratory, but on the wellspring of human motivation and action. They were about heart, compassion, knowledge (brain) and different concepts of suffering and the relative valuation of suffering. The caption to the *Lustiger Blätter* cartoon, if we reverse human and animal at every step, captures the argument of German (and English and American) medicine

---

[2] 'Die Vivisection des Meschen', *Lustiger Blätter*, 14:1 (1899): 8. My thanks to Lisa Hausofer for identifying the precise location and date of this source.

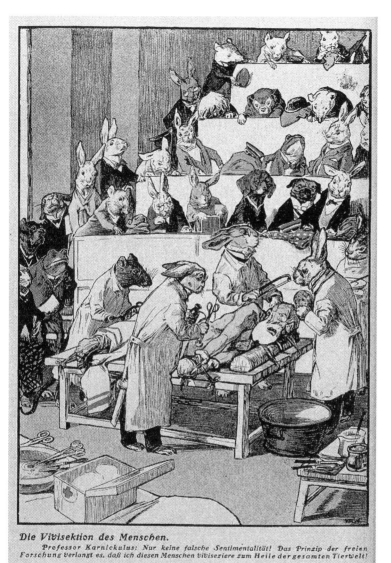

Die Vivisektion des Menschen.

Professor Karnickulus: Nur keine falsche Sentimentalität! Das Prinzip der freien Forschung verlangt es, daß ich diesen Menschen viviseziere zum Heile der gesamten Tierwelt!

Figure 2.2 'Die Vivisektion des Menschen', *Lustiger Blätter*, 1899. Wellcome Library London. Attribution 4.0 International (CC BY 4.0).

perfectly. It is to the context, and to the specific mobilization of that argument in the German-speaking countries, that I now turn.

Exported Ideas

Antivivisectionism quickly spread from England via Switzerland to Germany, the seat of experimental practice and physiological training.[3] It arrived fully formed, as it were, with the literature and strategies developed in the early 1870s being quickly translated for a local audience. Yet German scientists were not the same kind of target as English scientists. They were professional, highly specialized and employed by the State. Insofar as they expressed a strong commitment to scientific freedom, to pursue research as they saw fit, they did so as mandated by the State for the sake, at least nominally, of the common good. An attack on German science, therefore, was much more directly an attack on the German State than was ever the case in England. Indeed, the antivivisection movement in England had, in effect, implicated the State in the business of science in a novel way. For these reasons, antivivisectionism in Germany quickly took on a different form, becoming more radical and more consistently about animal ethics writ large, and, as such, it was far less dangerous to the freedom of scientists to practice as they pleased. Towards the end of the century, after significant failures in gaining any kind of parliamentary of legislative traction, German antivivisection would align itself more explicitly with anti-vaccination, naturopathy, vegetarianism, theosophy and anti-Semitism, making it, by 1900, something of a fringe pursuit.[4]

---

[3] I rely in this chapter on the timeline and framing of Ulrich Tröhler and Andreas-Holger Maehle, 'Anti-Vivisection in Nineteenth-Century Germany and Switzerland: Motives and Methods', *Vivisection in Historical Perspective*, ed. Nicolaas Rupke (London: Croom Helm, 1987), 149–87, but more acutely focus on the strategy and rhetoric of medical scientists. There are two book-length studies of antivivisection in Germany and environs, as well as one intellectual history of antivivisectionist ethics: H. Bretschneider, *Der Streit um die Vivisektion im 19. Jahrhundert. Verlauf – Argumente – Ergebnisse* (Stuttgart, 1962); Roland Neff, *Der Streit um den wissenschaftlichen Tierversuch in der Schweiz des 19. Jahrhunderts* (Basel: Schwabe, 1989); Monica Libell, *Morality beyond Humanity: Schopenhauer, Grysanowski, and Schweitzer on Animal Ethics* (Lund, 2001). For further context, see Andreas-Holger Maehle, 'The Ethical Discourse on Animal Experimentation, 1650–1900', in *Doctors and Ethics: The Earlier Historical Setting of Professional Ethics*, ed. A. Wear, J. Geyer-Kordesch and R. French, The Wellcome Series in the History of Medicine, Clio Medica, vol. 24 (Amsterdam, 1993); Andreas-Holger Maehle, 'Organisierte Tierversuchsgegner: Gründe und Grenzen ihrer gesellschaftlichen Wirkung, 1879–1933', in *Medizinkritische Bewegungen im Deutschen Reich (ca. 1870–ca. 1933)*, ed. M. Dinges, Medizin, Gesellschaft und Geschichte, suppl. vol. 9 (Stuttgart, 1996), 109–25.
[4] Tröhler and Maehle, 'Anti-Vivisection in Nineteenth-Century Germany', 174–8.

This being said, German scientists still felt troubled by the activities of antivivisectionists, and they still struck a defensive attitude. Yet in this period, the German scientific establishment did not immediately feel compelled to organize collectively, at least not to any great extent, to protect themselves. Their defence was as ad hoc as it was incoherent, perhaps reflective of the small extent to which they were troubled. More significantly, German scientists faced accusations outside of Germany of a brutality or callousness that was specific to the German national character. They were raised, by antivivisectionists and scientists alike, as being a dangerous influence on the morals and character of scientists in other countries. If there was callousness in experimental medicine, so one of the arguments went, it was not because the experiments themselves caused it, it was because Germanness was particularly vulnerable to moral numbness. Given that the rest of the civilized world was sending its brightest hopes for the medical future to Germany for training in experimental medicine, this perception of national character flaw was the cause of fear. What if, in the passing on of the best methods, techniques and knowledge, the German masters also passed on something of themselves? In this chapter I will sketch briefly the impact of antivivisectionism on German experimental science, and the response of some of Germany's most important researchers, but then turn the focus to the ways in which medical establishments in other countries negotiated the perceived risks of German contagion. How did they defend experimental medicine as a science while at the same time separating it from the personnel who, often by direct contact, had instructed them to do it?

German Experience

The story of the antivivisection movement in Germany is well enough known. Scant attention has been paid to scientific responses to it. This is, in part, because there was no organized defence on a grand scale. More important, perhaps, is the connection of the antivivisection movement in this period to later iterations of the same in Germany that came to be central to the National Socialist worldview. In between, the movement was attached to radical German political movements concerned with nature holism, which set it apart from its Anglophone counterpart. Whereas the relation in England with vegetarianism was always eschewed by the key antivivisection groups, the incorporation of antivivisection within a general form of nature worship was fuelled in Germany by the support of such luminaries as Richard Wagner (1813–83). That antivivisectionism in this period, everywhere, was a fundamentally *conservative* movement has escaped the notice of most of its historians, who have seen in it the radical underpinnings of modern animal rights politics and feminism. But at the heart of even the English movement was a concern about the abandonment of traditional feelings of a strictly Christian compassion, and of a re-ordering of social authority away from the church and towards the scientist. While it is reasonable enough to say that antivivisectionists were not anti-science through and through, they were nonetheless opposed to the vision of progress put forward by leading scientific researchers and their proponents. Moreover, they were deeply concerned with a shift in social authority from the pulpit to the laboratory. In Germany this was combined with another political strain that valorized nature and the human relation to it, that would also receive its most radical iteration under the Nazis. Antivivisection ended up as a core achievement of the Third Reich, and has thus baffled commentators who have tried to square an assumption of extended humanitarianism to animals with Nazi policies and practices concerning experimentation on those it considered subhuman.[5] This bafflement is based on a misunderstanding of the case, and of the central conservatism of antivivisectionism itself, but in the period under study here, all of this remained on the fringes of establishment thought and, barring a couple of flashpoints, outside of the mainstream of German politics. German science, especially the specialism of physiology, was world-leading and a source of pride. Attacks upon it, from abroad as well as from close at hand, were in general treated with dismay, disbelief and dismissal.

Given the extensive focus of English antivivisection agitation on German abuses, it is perhaps unsurprising that the movement was transplanted to Germany, where it was received by the German establishment as an unwelcome and distinctly alien presence. German scientists marvelled at the peculiar sensitivity of the English for the welfare of animals, and resented the lay public's interference in scientific matters. There was a mirroring of the English agitation in German antivivisection, which had a direct line to Frances Power Cobbe in particular. Ernst Grysanowski (1824–88), one of the principal German antivivisectionists, had had close contact with Cobbe in Italy, and was already primed about the antivivisectionist cause. He was further inspired by the manuscript of an antivivisectionist novel, sent to him for review by his friend Marie-Espérance von Schwartz (1818–99), and the two were launched into an antivivisectionist campaign, leaving Italy to realize their antivivisectionist writings back in Germany. The novel,

---

[5] Key work in this area has been undertaken by Boria Sax, who remains the leading scholar in understanding the manifold complexities of the status and meaning of 'animal' in the Third Reich. Boria Sax, *Animals in the Third Reich: Pets, Scapegoats, and the Holocaust* (New York: Continuum, 2000); Arnold Arluke and Boria Sax, 'Understanding Nazi Animal Protection and the Holocaust', *Anthrozoös*, 5 (1992): 6–31.

published pseudonymously under the name of Elpis Milena, was entitled *Gemma oder Tugend und Laster* [*Gemma or Virtue and Vice*] and appeared in English, French and Italian translations. It was this that caught the attention of the man who would transpire to be the movement's leader, Ernst von Weber (1830–1902).[6]

Von Weber observed in his *Torture Chambers of Science* how 'In England the conscience of the nation has … been awakened … and public opinion about the horrors of vivisection has forced a law to protect the unfortunate victims of this "scientific method of investigation" from the horrors of vivisection'. 'Should the German nation', he asked, 'fall behind the English?'[7] Indeed, the English, he said, had already 'led the European people in so many humanitarian directions', on questions of civil liberty, on the balance of public powers, on the social position of women, and on the emancipation of slaves. Vivisection was the obvious next step and he urged Germany to 'listen to the voice of humanity'.[8] He consistently and romantically associated public opinion in England with moral progress and, thinking specifically of Frances Power Cobbe, noted that

The fine-feeling noble Englishwoman tolerates in her society no man in whose raw soul the feelings of compassion and mercy are inaccessible, and in her eyes she gives noble and human feelings in man a much higher value than the mere dead mass of combined knowledge. Would that our German women, and our priests and teachers finally realise that the moral duty falls to them to raise a new generation of compassionate and merciful people.[9]

One notable scapegoat was Moritz Schiff (1823–96), who to the dissenting English moralist represented the worst possible example: a German scientist in Italy, or a callous operator in an immoral (Catholic) land. Freed from the moral scrutiny of the Italian public, which was represented consistently as indifferent to suffering, Schiff was at liberty, so it was reported, to torture animals at will.

The fear among some of the German-speaking medical establishment that an antivivisection movement might secure a footing at home was precipitated by the appointment of Schiff to the Chair of Physiology in Geneva in 1876, at the height of antivivisectionist attention in Britain. Pre-identified as a monstrous figure in the English press (see below), Schiff brought the prospect of horror much closer to home for Germans

---

[6] Tröhler and Maehle, 'Anti-Vivisection', 156–9. Elpis Milena [Marie-Espérance von Schwartz], *Gemma oder Tugend und Laster* (Franz, 1877); Iatros [Ernst Grysanowski], *Die Vivisektion, ihr wissenschaftlicher Wert und ihre ethische Berechtigung* (Leipzig, 1877).

[7] Ernst von Weber, *Die Folterkammern der Wissenschaft. Eine Sammlung von Thatsachen für das Laien-Publikum* (Berlin, 1879), n.p.

[8] Von Weber, *Die Folterkammern der Wissenschaft*, 5.

[9] Von Weber, *Die Folterkammern der Wissenschaft*, 65.

and German speakers. While Schiff himself sought to mollify, and while the Swiss establishment largely looked the other way, others saw the need to strike pre-emptively against the likelihood of a fully fledged antivivisection movement, lest Swiss and German science be taken off guard and subjected to regulatory control as had happened in Britain.

The most prolix of these was the Professor of Physiology at Zurich, Ludimar Hermann. His 1877 book *Die Vivisectionsfrage für das grössere Publicum beleuchtet* was an extended review of the controversy in England, the parliamentary inquiry, the impacts on scientific freedom, and the unthinkable prospect of a clash between the principles of humanity held up by animal protection societies and the scientific establishment. Crucially, Hermann identified from the outset the tremendous risk of a campaign against medical and scientific research that appealed to emotion above evidence:

> The feelings [*Gefühle*] that the prosecutors call in reverberate powerfully in every breast, and the object is ripe for the negligent or deliberate dissemination of false or exaggerated statements, so that the truth would have no chance of fighting its own way. Almost none of the agitators, let alone the majority, has seen a physiological experiment – very few tried to get an idea of it by reading physiological works.

Implicit in his complaint was that the public at large had no prior knowledge of what went on in physiological laboratories and were, by this agitation, only becoming misled, misinformed and emotionally manipulated. Popular protestors, he said, were like children, shedding tears over an unhappy fairy tale. They were people who had gone from complete ignorance of a science called physiology to, a moment later, grief and indignation at the crimes committed daily in institutions maintained by the state, by people in the state's employ.[10] Against this sentimentality they presented the callous physiologist and his students, hearts hardened by the sight of tortured animals. Hermann waved this away impatiently, suggesting that if it were true it would have to apply also to the medical student in his encounter with the sick, or in the preparation of corpses. Of course, such arguments had been made many times before, but implicit here was an appeal to the *delicacy* or tenderness [*Zartgefühl*] of men involved in medical research, in an overall context of awareness-raising.[11] Hermann called the 1876 Act in England 'one of the strangest . . . of all time', and complained that from 'inconspicuous beginnings in Florence, the agitation against vivisection . . . found such wonderfully favourable ground [in England] that in a very short time it

---

[10] Ludimar Hermann, *Die Vivisectionsfrage für das grössere Publicum beleuchtet* (Leipzig: Vogel, 1877), 3–4.
[11] Hermann, *Die Vivisectionsfrage*, 25–6.

celebrated a complete triumph over science'. This was the result of 'tender souls' like Richard Hutton, editor of *The Spectator* and member of the Royal Commission, who represented physiology as 'evil', and who filled his report with 'emotional paragraphs' about cats and dogs.[12] We will turn to Hutton shortly. 'In no time', Hermann complained, 'men who had the confidence to participate in beneficent ways in the great objectives of promoting human knowledge ... are referred to the dock, accused of trampling one of the most beautiful of human feelings: compassion for helpless creatures'.[13] On the contrary, it was, he claimed, precisely a more refined, more civilized compassion that activated physiologists. If sensitivity to pain was a marker of the civilized individual, then their actions to alleviate the suffering of the many while rigidly adhering to the administration of anaesthetics in their operations surely indicated their own highly civilized status.

If Hermann was the most fulsome in his complaints, Tröhler and Maehle nevertheless count twenty-one publications in favour of vivisection in German between 1877 and 1883, matching a peak of output in these years in Britain. They mostly ensued from the pens of those invested in medical research and who played a part of the medical establishment. There were many more publications against them, including translations of English pamphlets and a concerted attempt to convert animal protection societies in Germany to the antivivisectionist cause, the very thing Hermann had thought 'unthinkable'. One notable piece in support of vivisection came from the pen of Carl Ludwig (1816–95), a giant in the field of physiology and founder of the Physiological Institute in Leipzig (Figure 2.3).[14] Ludwig was also a vice-president of the animal welfare association in Leipzig, representing a major block to antivivisectionist ambitions. Ludwig, according to Monica Libell, 'took great precautions to minimize animal suffering and lectured his colleagues and students about ... the importance of using anaesthetics. The vivisectionists, Ludwig maintained, were "the true friends of both man and animal", and their position made them well equipped to value the suffering of the vivisected animals'.[15] Ludwig published his response to the antivivisectionists in *Die Gartenlaube*, a popular magazine, to maximize his impact with a lay audience. He reflected on the relation of the vivisection controversy to English medicine's lack of a formal relation to the State, and he bemoaned what he saw as the English clergy's imposition of its own values onto matters it did not understand. 'Just as the Popes feared that Copernicus and his disciple Galileo would be the destroyers of

---

[12] Hermann, *Die Vivisectionsfrage*, 48.   [13] Hermann, *Die Vivisectionsfrage*, 4.
[14] W. Bruce Fye, 'Carl Ludwig and the Leipzig Physiological Institute: "A Factory of New Knowledge"', *Circulation*, 74 (1986): 920–28.
[15] Libell, *Morality beyond Humanity*, 241–3.

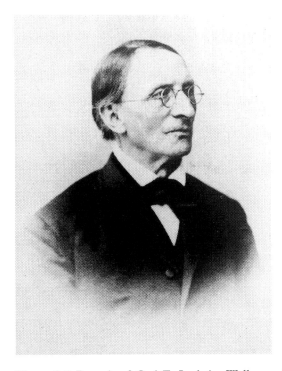

Figure 2.3 Portrait of Carl F. Ludwig. Wellcome Library, London. Attribution 4.0 International (CC BY 4.0).

the traditional heavens', he wrote, 'so the English clergy imagines that physiology can alienate the soul'. He determined to prove the 'eminent degree of humanity' and the 'scientific benefits' of vivisection.[16]

Ernst von Weber, seeing the futility of appropriating the existing animal welfare organizations, so long as men like Ludwig were involved in them, established his own animal protection society (Der Neue Leipziger Thierschutzverein) in Leipzig in 1879, specifically to institutionalize the fight against animal research. At its launch, Ludwig's piece in *Die Gartenlaube* became the focus of Weber's scorching inaugural speech, in which von Weber indulged in the themes he had explored in *The Torture Chambers of Science*. It caused a stir. Weber gave an extraordinary speech to the respectable audience on the subject of vivisection from a moral stand-point, calling Ludwig's article a 'Meisterstück der Sophistik' – a masterpiece

---

[16] C. Ludwig, 'Die "Vivisection" vor dem Richterstuhl der Gegenwart: Ein Wort zur Vermittelung', *Die Gartenlaube* (1879): 417–19.

of sophistry – and railing against the practice of vivisection. But at the close of the meeting, somebody from the floor proposed an ovation to Ludwig, and the crowd moved in droves to the street to express in high voice their love and reverence for, as the Leipzig press put it, a most venerated man. Thus an evening designed for the vilification of Ludwig by his enemies ended in celebration of the same man.[17] A few days later, the front page of the *Leipziger Tageblatt* ran with a long and searing editorial on the vivisection question, leaving no question where respectable opinion ought to lie. The argument ran thus: if at that moment it was the physicians against whom hatred was poured in public, then at the next moment it would be the clergy, military officers and the judges against whom misguided heads would turn. It was, in the opinion of this newspaper, the duty of all who clung to the state as the haven of their existence to assemble against these anti-societal agitations and put them down, lest society be lost to the enemies of social order.[18]

Ludwig's article, Weber's event, and the press analysis of it are indicative of why antivivisection never attained the reach or influence in Germany that it did in Britain or the USA. First, scientific research was carried out under the auspices of the State, and there had been considerable investment over the previous couple of decades in Germany in making sure that the State was an object of virtue or veneration in the eyes of the public. It could, so the argument went, be trusted. Second, physiology was incorporated into mainstream understandings of *humanity* from the beginning, with no apparent dissonance between a respectable and progressive animal welfare movement and scientific research. The argument was still rehearsed, but how much easier was it to rehearse it with the welfare societies already on board?[19] Third, at a popular level, men of science were local and national heroes, embodiments of the State, in fact. Ludwig's name was cheered on the streets by his students, who curried favour with a public that knew plenty about the man, his character, his fame and reputation.

Still, these events, and the availability of von Weber's *Torture Chambers of Science*, seem to have inspired Ludwig, who initiated what might be thought of as the first coordinated strategy to defend animal experimentation in Germany and Switzerland. This is documented by Maehle and

---

[17] 'Neuer Leipziger Thierschutzverein', *Zweite Beilage zum Leipziger Tageblatt und Anzeiger*, 4 December 1879.

[18] 'Die Angriffe des Herrn v. Weber auf Vivisectoren und Aerzte', *Erste Beilage zum Leipziger Tageblatt und Anzeiger*, 8 December 1879.

[19] Tröhler and Maehle, 'Anti-Vivisection', describe the mollification of Swiss animal welfarists (152–3) as well as pointing out the sharp distinction between German antivivisection societies and German animal welfare societies. There were 'less than a dozen' of the former, in c. 1900, among 150 general welfare societies, and the members of the radical groups were often formally excluded from the more moderate mainstream, which acknowledged the potential utility of animal research (179).

Tröhler, so I will recount it in brief.[20] A circular letter was issued from Leipzig, enclosed with a copy of von Weber's pamphlet, and sent to twenty-six medical faculties across Germany and Switzerland, requesting their joint signature on a declaration concerning the positive benefits of animal experimentation for advances in medical science, which was to be published in the major newspapers. Indeed, medical progress was argued to be predicated on vivisection. Maehle and Tröhler note that sixteen faculties had joined their signature to the declaration within a month, but it is in the response of those which refused that we find the essential character of the German situation. To respond publicly risked 'attracting the attention of the public', and it was none of their concern. In Berlin in particular, there was an expression of confidence that the Prussian Ministry of Culture would favour 'the interests of science', which the scientists would argue were identical with the best interests of public health (where expert opinion was deemed to carry far more weight than popular opinion). Why risk inflaming an already sore point by engaging with it? Science was not to be gauged in the court of popular opinion, but could only be weighed by the expertise of professionals in the employ of the State.

Wherever German scientists did engage directly with public opinion, therefore, this broader context of confidence, falling back on a trust in governmental support, must be taken into account. It allowed men such as Rudolf Heidenhain (1834–97) to emphasize the risk to German science through the otherworldliness of English antivivisection. It was not medical research that had been corrupted, but the emotional bearing of the general public, whose general lack of education seemed no longer to hold them back on making sentimental pronouncements on things beyond their ken. Heidenhain was Chair of Physiology at Breslau, whose students included Ivan Pavlov (1849–1936). He was bewildered by what he saw as a strange English humanity. 'The English nation has never before shied away from brazenly kicking people to crush them, where there was a material interest', he said. Humanitarianism there was a sham, a mere gloss on an otherwise brutal imperialism, and now fixed on the pain of animals. For Heidenhain, it was a smokescreen. 'From where', he asked, 'for those who consider it permissible to sacrifice millions of human beings for the purpose of accumulating the riches of the world in Great Britain, from where comes the deep feeling for the animal that disturbances to the thirst for knowledge and the promotion and mastery of the knowledge of natural laws are day by day threatening the health and life of the people?' He suggested that it was time physiologists were roused from their laboratories, and that, lest they succumb to the

---

[20] Tröhler and Maehle, 'Anti-Vivisection', 166.

example of the English, they should educate the lay public in the achievements of physiology and the humanitarian goals for which it strove.[21] His educative impulse was a minority one among German scientists. Why struggle to inform the masses, who might never fully understand the justifications of experiments, given the expertise it took to design them and carry them out? Better, surely, to leave them in the dark.

Antivivisectionists tried to plead their case before German legislatures both regional and national. Insofar as they found support, they found it among conservative politicians whose knowledge did not extend beyond what was written in antivivisectionist propaganda. Yet they met resistance in the form of medical expertise embedded in the political fabric. Rudolf Virchow, the renowned Berlin pathologist and physician, happened also to be a liberal member of the Reichstag and was able to thwart early attempts, in 1880, to petition the national government to act with respect to regulating the practice of vivisection.

The following year, Virchow addressed the IMC in the heat of antivivisectionist ire in London, having left a blossoming antivivisection movement in Leipzig and Dresden that was beginning to register in Berlin. His address in London distanced him, in certain respects, from his allies in England (as did his opposition to Darwinism), but it did establish the terms upon which vivisection would be represented on a formal, political stage back in Germany. Virchow expressed the absurdity of a moral calculus in which torture was deemed worse than death, comparing vivisection tacitly to legal punishment. What kind of system would aver that the death penalty were less severe than mere torture? He could not understand, in his analogy, why antivivisectionists would insist that a vivisected animal could not emerge from the anaesthesia and make a recovery. Why kill it, as if death were a mere trifle, and torture were the worst of ordeals?[22] Here he badly underestimated the extent to which suffering dominated the debate in England, but he was not alone in Germany in voicing such an opinion. Friedrich Goltz, for example, boasted that 'It was important ... that the dogs from which [he] had, for example, removed pieces of the brain, had their lives saved and were healed.'[23] The survival of the animal was aided by the use of anaesthesia in the operation. Here was the major bone of contention in Ferrier's trial, in which Goltz was clearly implicated. English scientists, the Ferrier/Yeo experiments notwithstanding, would argue that the whole utility of

[21] Rudolf Heidenhain, *Die Vivisection im Dienste der Heilkunde*, 2nd edn (Leipzig, 1879), 5.
[22] Rudolf Virchow, 'An Address on the Value of Pathological Experiments', *BMJ*, 6 (1881): 198–203.
[23] Friedrich Goltz, *Wider die Humanaster. Rechtfertigung eines Vivisektors* (Strassburg, 1883), 5–6.

anaesthesia would be undone by allowing the animal to regain consciousness. The effects of suffering on the animal were inversely reflected in the vivisectors' capacity to endure or even overlook that suffering, such that Virchow's comments (and those of Goltz) would have seemed to many to confirm the kind of monstrousness that he was endeavouring to deny. Yet, for all that Virchow tried to couch his defence of experiment in terms of a moral code that might be readily understood by a layman, it was ultimately to a mark of distinction from the layman that he appealed. For a man 'who has a greater interest in domestic animals than in science, that is, in the knowledge of truth, is not qualified to be an official controller of scientific affairs'.[24] No inspector of experimental research could possibly be recruited from without scientific bowers. Independence equalled ignorance. 'To what would it lead', Virchow asked rhetorically, 'if an experimenter, who had commenced his experiment in good faith, had perhaps to answer to some layman during the experiment, or to a magistrate afterwards, the charge that he had not selected some other method, or some other instruments, or perhaps some other experiment?'[25]

It was the expertise and experience of the experimenter that safeguarded experiments from excess. Though little was made of this etymological overlap – expertise, experience, experiment – these categories afforded the scientist an impenetrably circular logic of exclusion.[26] Without having personally *undergone* the procedure of research, which is to say, without being personally implicated in the methods of knowledge production, nobody could win the right to comment on the ethics of the procedure. To know, or to come to know, was implicitly entangled with science conceived as a verb. It had to be done, made, practised. Curiosity coupled with existing knowledge and technique led to new knowledge and new techniques, which in turn fostered more. One could not simply enter into the middle of an experimental procedure and pronounce on its ethics or its logic or its justification. For German scientists, as employees of the State, this position was even easier to maintain. The professional distance it gave them made the outrage of the public seem misplaced at best.

Virchow spelled this out in condescending terms. The 'outraged feelings of the possessor of horses, pet dogs, and parlour cats' are excited by a 'belief that the same thing may happen to his beloved animals as to the animals in the learned institute'. Virchow could 'sympathise' with this, but he offered assurances that nobody would be compelled to 'deliver to us his favourites,

---

[24] Virchow, 'An Address', 203.   [25] Virchow, 'An Address', 203.
[26] For the general context of this connection, see Rob Boddice, ed., *Scientific and Medical Knowledge Production, 1796–1918: Experiment, Expertise, Experience*, 4 vols (London: Routledge, forthcoming).

nor would we steal them'.[27] This kind of sentimental objection to experimental research was a flight of fancy, disconnected from anything to do with science itself. It was understandable, perhaps, but utterly ignorant nonetheless. Scientists, he espoused, 'should not be considered or declared to be *à priori* rough, void of moral feelings, and barbarians standing almost on the threshold of crime'. There was, he said, no 'evidence that moral earnestness is failing in modern medical circles'. To say that 'Christianity is imperilled by vivisection' was 'worthy of Abdera', the famous city ridiculed for its stupidity. The 'assertion that the medical youth are inevitably "brutalised" by dissection and vivisection, is, as usual, snatched from the air; as it is also a calumny that the vivisection teachers have suffered injury to their morality'.[28] All such slogans came from outside of scientific experience, experience that could only be gained through practice. The volume of the outcry was matched only by its irrelevance. Virchow's 'expression of the freedom of science' was that 'the carrying out of the experiment must remain in his [the scientist's] own hands'.[29] Science was like the sun in Bacon's *Novum Organum*: it shone on palaces and sewers alike, but was not thereby polluted. For all that the masses might complain in their stinking ignorance, science was undimmed.

Such a view might have been entertained with a certain satisfaction among men of the same standing, but it can hardly be thought to have been an effective strategy for winning hearts and minds beyond the profession. Indeed, Virchow's aloofness would have indicated precisely that roughness of which he said scientists took no share. While such views provided German scientists the wherewithal to put their heads down and carry on with their work, the token sympathy for the concerns of the general public for the welfare of their 'parlour cats' smelled strongly of the callousness that the same public feared could easily be magnified into monstrousness. The fact that Virchow made his speech in London, where he was feted by English scientists, made the threat of German contagion there seem tangible.

Back in the Reichstag in 1882, Virchow picked up his thread from London and expounded upon it, denouncing lay abuse based on half knowledge and anecdote in the name of shackling the freedom of scientific research. The refusal of the national government to entertain legislation against vivisection at this point effectively nipped the matter in the bud, at least as far as antivivisection represented a national threat to German science.[30] Physiological research was already the business of the German State; its dismissal of antivivisectionism ensured the status quo.

[27] Virchow, 'An Address', 203.   [28] Virchow, 'An Address', 203.
[29] Virchow, 'An Address', 203.   [30] Tröhler and Maehle, 'Anti-Vivisection', 167–8.

On a local level, things were somewhat more protracted. In Prussia, a petition from the radical antivivisection animal protection societies in 1883 was underscored by Ernst von Weber's engineering of the debate such as to co-opt not only Richard Wagner (who was certainly an antivivisectionist, but in a politics of nature holism that can hardly be described as mainstream) and Bismarck himself.[31] The result of the ensuing parliamentary commission was therefore different to the outcome in the Reichstag, despite the efforts of Virchow to stall the petition. Yet the process of formal enquiry was drawn out and ended up in a government endorsement of the status quo, inspired in part by the fact that the vast majority of German animal protection societies refused to sign on to von Weber's radical campaign and by an uptick in scientific representations of experimental practices and their moral and social value. Gustav von Gossler (1838–1902), the Prussian Minister of Education, had conducted the enquiry and also commissioned a new work by Rudolf Heidenhain, which was published in 1884.[32]

Heidenhain thus became a kind of figurehead for German science insofar as the establishment saw any need to communicate with, or justify itself to, the general public. His 1884 work, despite acknowledging the fact that it was commissioned by the Prussian government in the very title, nonetheless opened with a declaration that it had been carried out with a view to the undecided layman, projecting an argument about the centrality and essential quality of vivisection for the progress of science. What followed was fairly typical for the genre in both England and the USA, but was markedly unusual in the German context. Heidenhain laid out the history of knowledge produced by vivisection that could not have been produced by any other means, and coupled it with the procedural, therapeutic and pharmaceutical benefits of this knowledge. It was a greatest-hits of medical discovery and progress, from angina pectoris to wound infections, from trichinosis to aseptic surgery, with hopes expressed for the cure of such spectres as cholera, all derived from animal experimentation. Heidenhain went on to justify the repetition of experiments (those who criticized such repetitions did not understand the nature of science) and denied, in a quite extraordinary manner given the aim of his book to reach a lay audience, the capacity of laymen to assess the practices and justifications of vivisection, and physiology in particular.[33] Criticism from without was bound to be wrong since it

---

[31] Ernst von Weber, *Bisher ungedruckte Briefe von Richard Wagner an Ernst von Weber* (Dresden, 1883).

[32] Rudolf Heidenhain, *Die Vivisection. Auf Veranlassung des Königlich Preußischen Ministers der geistlichen, Unterrichts- und Medicinal- Angelegenheiten* (Leipzig: Breitkopf and Härtel, 1884); Tröhler and Maehle, 'Anti-Vivisection', 169–70.

[33] Heidenhain, *Die Vivisection*, 49.

lacked the specialist expertise required for a formal assessment. This, logically, ought also to have ruled out praise from the layman, but the rhetorical inconsistency did not register. Trust, therefore, was the guiding principle, which justified the practice of vivisection as none of the public's business, coupled with the claim that the public could not have understood it even if it were. Heidenhain's book is exemplary of a genre that would blossom in England and in the USA over the next three decades, at the same time extolling the virtues of medical progress by experimentation and denying the public any capacity to know or understand this beyond a pithy balance-sheet of the benefits derived for mankind against negligible pains in the other column. The kicker, the perennial get-out-jail-free argument, was that most science was conducted without any immediate utility for human life. It simply was not the motivation for science, even if it was often the outcome. No experiment could be judged, before the fact, on the knowledge it would produce or on the benefits that would derive from it, because these were the *results* of experiment, the *results* of experience.[34] Science was about the pursuit and production of knowledge, activated by curiosity. Humanity was inherent to such curiosity because it was already known that the experimental method did tend towards 'progress', and a lack of useful results did not negate this general truth.

To this was coupled a series of appendices that drew on international encounters with antivivisection and the responses of the medical establishment in Germany and other countries, including the declaration signed by medical faculties in Germany, Austria and Switzerland that had been initiated by Ludwig, a bibliography of works by German scientists that supported the line of argument put forward by Heidenhain, the declaration of the IMC in 1881, the declaration of the British Medical Association of the same year, the memorandum of the AAMR, and a Resolution of the Medical Society of the State of New York.[35]

In the meantime, Gossler had sent a circular letter to the German Medical Faculties containing eleven questions and asking them to self report. The questions asked about the indispensability of the experimental method to both research and teaching, its scale and the nature of its practice, as well as any knowledge of abuses. The answers, which came in from Berlin, Bonn, Breslau, Göttingen, Greifswald, Halle, Kiel, Königsberg and Marburg, universally and ringingly endorsed vivisection. The faculty at Berlin, for example, asserted that any inroads into the freedom to conduct experimental research would lead to

---

[34] Heidenhain, *Die Vivisection*, 49.   [35] Heidenhain, *Die Vivisection*, 91ff.

'absolute paralysis of Medical Science and the annihilation of its further progress'.[36]

With such an array of authorities and expertise, Gossler felt safe to let the matter drop in Prussia, decreeing that animal experimentation could continue as before, without any significant let or hindrance. Faced with anger in the Prussian Landtag, Gossler and Virchow rallied on this question of expertise and medical authority and, according to Maehle and Tröhler, 'marked the political defeat for decades to come of Ernst von Weber and his group'.[37] The question of the ethics of experimentation and the need for regulation did not go away, but the need for a strategic defence of vivisection in Germany and environs ceased by the mid 1880s, decades earlier than in England or the USA. When the problem did come back, in the first years of the new century, the worst fears of antivivisectionists seemed to have been realized: humans were the new experimental animals. I reserve an account of this for the epilogue to this volume.

German Spectres

If German antivivisection looked to England for inspiration, English scientists gazed in turn upon their German colleagues with admiration. Into the 1860s, the established medical-scientific community in Britain still adhered to the principles of the amateur generalist, and insofar as there was an experimental or investigative impetus, it took place in the morbid field of anatomy, where the object of study was dead: to begin with. If travel to, and . education in, German academic institutions was by no means new by the 1870s, it was nonetheless a growing phenomenon, and the importation of physiology was a significant novelty that rapidly altered the research priorities of British medical science.[38] The beginning of this movement coincided with the publication of *The Handbook for the Physiological Laboratory*, which wore its debt to continental and particularly to German physiology quite openly, raising fears that European callousness had, in fact, already arrived.[39]

---

[36] Gossler's decree, and the replies to his circular letter, were translated and issued as a pamphlet by the AAMR in 1885. On this occasion, German medical justifications met the approval of English scientists: *Official Circular Addressed to the German Universities by the Minister of Public Instruction Enjoining Safeguards against Abuses of Vivisection, with an Appendix Containing the Statements of the Several Medical Faculties* (London: J. W. Kolckmann, 1885), quote p. 5.

[37] Tröhler and Maehle, 'Anti-Vivisection', 170.

[38] For the prior generation of scientific exchange with Germany, see John Davis, 'Higher Education Reform and the German Model: A Victorian Discourse', in *Anglo-German Scholarly Networks in the Long Nineteenth Century*, ed. Heather Ellis and Ulrike Kirchberger (Leiden: Brill, 2014).

[39] The *Handbook*'s debt to German research is clearly laid out in Stewart Richards, 'Drawing the Life-Blood of Physiology', 33–9, esp. 37.

The outcry at what was represented to be Schiff's dog-torturing laboratory in Florence was, strangely, the beginning of the antivivisection
movement in England. The English moral campaigner Frances Power
Cobbe – in Florence acting as correspondent for the *Daily News*
(London) – first alerted the public to it in 1863.[40] The perceived distance
of Schiff's activities from daily goings on in English science perhaps
accounts for the initial failure of the story to take hold to any great degree.
A decade later, however, experimental physiology was an emerging force,
especially at University College, London, and Schiff's activities were re-
examined in this light.[41]

The story was picked up by Richard Hutton, the editor of the *Spectator*
magazine. Hutton was among the loudest antivivisectionists, as well as
being distinctly suspicious of German morals in the context of medical
science. He was to serve on the committee of the Royal Commission, and
was responsible for much of the anti-German tenor of the inquiry. As is the
case for many of the participants in the controversy, it is not possible to paint
Hutton as a thoroughgoing anti-German. He had himself studied in
Heidelberg and Berlin in the 1840s, and repeatedly returned for holidays,
appropriating, to a certain degree, a German manner in his personal affect-
ations. In the 1850s, G. H. Lewes accused him of being overly influenced by
German aesthetic criticism in his popular reviews for the *Spectator*. Yet for
all his experience Hutton ran an anti-Kaiser, as well as an antivivisectionist,
newspaper, and he remained suspicious of Germans at the level of the heart.
He once expressed dismay at 'various kinds of sentiment – for which, thank
God, we have no terms in our language' going on explicitly to condemn 'the
expansiveness of French "effusion" and the sickly conceit of German
"Gefühl" [which] have no kindred with genuine feeling'. The criticism
was literary, but it spilled over into his general ethics.[42]

---

[40] For Cobbe's involvement in antivivisection in general, see Rob Boddice, *A History of
Attitudes and Behaviours toward Animals in Eighteenth- and Nineteenth-Century Britain:
Anthropocentrism and the Emergence of Animals* (Lewiston, NY: Mellen, 2009), 326–33.

[41] For more on Schiff's activities in Florence, see Patrizia Guarnieri, 'Moritz Schiff'.

[42] Details of Hutton's general attitude towards Germany are compiled from
Malcolm Woodfield, 'Victorian Weekly Reviews and Reviewing after 1860: R.H.
Hutton and the *Spectator*', *The Yearbook of English Studies*, 16 (1986): 74–91, esp. 83;
Robert A. Colby, '"How It Strikes a Contemporary": The "Spectator" as Critic',
Nineteenth-Century Fiction, 11 (1956): 182–206, esp. 195; Gaylord C. Leroy, 'Richard
Holt Hutton', *PMLA*, 56 (1941): 809–40, esp. 814. The mistrust of the Kaiser occasionally spilled over into a general unease. Asking, in 1871, whether German 'cultivation'
would be any guarantee that Germany would be an 'Empire of Peace', the *Spectator*'s
editorial opined: 'where is the proof that culture is a guarantee for moderation? No
culture can surpass that of the German Professorate [sic], which throughout the last
seven years has been more exacting in its requirements, more hostile to other nations,
more completely penetrated with the spirit of dominance than either the people or the
soldiery of Germany' (*Spectator*, 44 [1871]: 341).

Taking up the outrage of Schiff's vivisection in Florence, Hutton reported in the *Spectator* that the eminent physiologist 'did not scruple to make Florence ring with the screams of his living subjects', and that this should sound a 'warning to English physiologists of the loathsome insensibility to which the habit of vivisection is apt to lead'. 'Professor Schiff', said Hutton, 'represents the most hideous depth of human hard-heartedness'.[43]

The prominent English zoologist, biologist and physiologist E. Ray Lankester (1847–1929) responded angrily in the pages of the *Spectator*. Ray Lankester was raised in the bosom of science, being introduced to Darwin, Huxley and others as a boy. Having taken first-class honours in natural sciences at Oxford, Ray Lankester won the Radcliffe travelling fellowship and took himself to the continent, studying physiology at Leipzig and Vienna, and morphology with Ernst Haeckel (1834–1919) at Jena, before finding another prominent German scientist in Italy, Anton Dohrn (1840–1909), with whom he studied marine zoology in Naples.[44] He was representative of the young English physiologist, who commonly felt the need to seek the leading German scientists in order to complete his education. Ray Lankester dismissed the 'exaggerated gossip' surrounding Schiff, whom he knew to be 'a humane and kind-hearted man', and 'one of the six most eminent physiologists of Europe'. The humanity of the physiologist was the key point for Ray Lankester, who insisted that vivisectors 'have not become callous to the sufferings of animals'. On the contrary, the 'experimenter often suffers most acutely from his sympathy with the animal, but controls his emotion and endures his pain in companionship with the dumb animal for the sake of science'.[45] This would become a keynote of physiological arguments, that the medical scientist was not only humane per se, but knew how to control his sympathy in the context of the laboratory for the sake of a greater good.

Among the members of the Royal Commission, Hutton of the *Spectator* was principally responsible for raising the question of the moral influence of German methods. He asked leading questions about the distinction between German, or 'Continental' methods, and English morals, hoping to be able to show the degradation of the latter through the influence of the former. He found encouragement with the representative of the Royal Society for the Prevention of Cruelty to Animals, who feared the importation of 'Continental usages' into England, but also with the older members of the

---

[43] *Spectator*, 46 (1873): 1643.
[44] Peter J. Bowler, 'Lankester, Sir (Edwin) Ray (1847–1929)', in *Oxford Dictionary of National Biography* (Oxford: Oxford University Press, 2004), online edn, www.oxforddnb.com/view/article/34406, accessed 1 February 2012.
[45] *Spectator*, 47 (1874): 13–14.

scientific establishment, who had had little direct experience with Germany.[46]

He asked James Paget, the eminent pathologist who would become a key member of the AAMR, whether 'our own medical men' 'come back with these new methods in their heads' from the schools in Leipzig, Vienna, Paris and Florence, and Paget assured him that 'Nothing imported from any of the schools you mention is commonly employed in the schools here', but then he had to admit that he knew nothing about the experiments carried out in any of those places.[47] That claim was scarcely credible. Similarly, Hutton pressed William Sharpey, whose career was spent bridging the disciplines of anatomy and physiology, about the 'natural effect of the very large study of our physiologists', especially in Germany, and Sharpey confessed that the influence of a place like Leipzig would naturally alter the methods used on the return to England.[48] The evolutionary biologist George Rolleston worried that physiology was being reduced to mere vivisection, and pointed out that each of Schiff's lectures in particular had 'some animal sacrificed for it'.[49] Henry Acland (1815–1900), Regius Professor of Medicine at Oxford and President of the General Medical Council, went further, calling the quest for knowledge through the study of living beings 'a new phase in modern thought' which brought into question the 'nature of our whole being and moral responsibilities'. Acland, although he confessed he had not visited the continental laboratories in question, nevertheless averred that 'things were done ... habitually' in them that 'would not be tolerated' in England. Continental science was carried on with 'unscientific careless-ness' that would be 'hurtful to the moral sense of England'. He was, however, reassured that 'the public feeling in England secures the English community against the infliction of purposeless and uncalled for suffering upon living animals'.[50] Michael Foster, who, unusually for an influential physiologist, had no direct experience outside of England, shared that sentiment, declaring his faith in the durability of 'the good feeling which characterizes the Englishmen who have taken part' in the experimental method of the Continent.[51] But it was a point of contention. The Rev. Samuel Haughton (1821–97), medical registrar of the School of Physic of Trinity College, Dublin, lamented the 'unnecessary and clumsy repetitions' of experiments reported in German journals, by young physi-ologists in England who made a point of learning German. 'There is

[46] Royal Commission on Vivisection, 82.   [47] Royal Commission on Vivisection, 16–17.
[48] Royal Commission on Vivisection, 27.   [49] Royal Commission on Vivisection, 68.
[50] Royal Commission on Vivisection, 43, 47–8.
[51] Royal Commission on Vivisection, 128–9.

a good deal of that second rate sort of physiological practice going on', he said, adding 'All of that . . . requires control'.[52]

The attitude among the older generation of establishment scientists and medical researchers might best be summarized as an informed reflection of the doubts raised by lay public opinion. It was not only that German ethics were treated with some circumspection, but that German scientific practices were embedded in a professionalized and specialized institution that answered to the State. The observation that young English physiologists were now finishing their educations on the Continent therefore allowed for the bundling of a cluster of latent fears within the scientific establishment. Put simply, the concern was that the German moral economy of physiology would be imported along with German apparatus and German methods.

Among the younger scientists who testified there was much greater circumspection about denouncing Germanic sensibilities. Philip Henry Pye-Smith had spent 'time abroad in Vienna and Berlin, forming what proved to be lasting friendships with Professor Virchow and others', before becoming lecturer on physiology at Guy's hospital.[53] Pye-Smith found himself unable to extend his view that there were 'no abuses for which correction would be desirable' to all countries, but he did not elaborate.[54] His colleague, F. W. Pavy (1829–1911), who had borne witness to the experiments of Claude Bernard (1813–78) in Paris in the 1850s, concurred that 'more is done in other countries than is done here' that would transgress the 'sentiment . . . of the medical profession'.[55] But he was certain that English students were too sensitive to withstand any exhibition of callousness, and always sought to assure them that 'no experiment will be introduced which will wound the feelings of the most sensitive amongst them'. Pavy's sentiments were echoed by Drs Rutherford and McDonnell (1828–89), of Edinburgh and Dublin respectively, and supported by Sir William Gull, who assured the committee that 'anything like cruelty or indifference to suffering would be scouted by the public opinion of the students'.[56] As a rule, most of the scientists who testified before the Commission did not see the necessity of repeating experiments for the sake of demonstration, and physiological neophytes tended to be guided through the experimental method by the close supervision of an expert. Doubts about the impersonal nature of German lecture-based teaching that applied in other fields were

---

[52] Royal Commission on Vivisection, 100.
[53] 'Philip Henry Pye-Smith, M.D., F.R.C.P., F.R.S'., *BMJ*, 1 (1914): 1215 (published 30 May 1914).
[54] Royal Commission on Vivisection, 109.   [55] Royal Commission on Vivisection, 109.
[56] Royal Commission of Vivisection, Report, x.

therefore somewhat mitigated in the case of physiology, but as we have seen, men like Huxley saw a great risk in limiting teaching capacities in this way.[57]

Another student of Bernard's, John Burdon Sanderson, led the physiological revolution at University College, an institution that had had close connections with the German academic world from its inception.[58] He was editor and co-author (with Michael Foster, Emanuel Klein and T. Lauder Brunton) of the *Handbook for the Physiological Laboratory*. Burdon Sanderson confessed that although the subject of physiology was 'founded to the extent of about perhaps nine parts out of ten upon experiments conducted in foreign countries', that there were nevertheless 'things done ... abroad ... which ought not to be done on humanitarian grounds'. He was sure that the 'sentiment is quite different among physiological workers' in England, and that this inevitably influenced the way in which physiology was practised. Still, Burdon Sanderson lauded German science. Hutton asked him if he wished to see 'the education here more like the type of education in Germany', to which Burdon Sanderson replied that he did 'not want to introduce any German institutions because they are German, but simply because they are efficient'. In a roundabout way, he expressed confidence in the 'reasonable humanity' of the 'leading men in Germany', and praised the methodological exactness there, where, he said, 'exactness is really more valued than it is in France'.[59]

Part of the problem for the British physiologists who had finished their training in Germany lay in convincing the Commission that Englishmen would not go to the same experimental lengths as the Germans, even though they had directly requested that their German peers instruct them in physiology through the fullness of the experimental method. Edward Schäfer of University College, who had German roots and had studied in Ludwig's laboratory in Leipzig, suggested that the eminence of the physiologist conducting an experiment – and here he singled out Ludwig in particular – generally meant that the experiment did not need to be repeated in England.[60] Arthur Gamgee (1841–1909), professor of physiology at Owens College, Manchester, concurred. He had studied with Wilhelm Kühne (1837–1900) at Heidelberg, and with Ludwig in Leipzig in 1871, and claimed to know 'foreign' physiologists 'pretty intimately'. He proclaimed Ludwig to be a man 'as cautious in the performance of any experiment on a living animal as any English physiologist that ever lived, and who yet has been the teacher of nearly all the physiologists of Europe, and has indoctrinated nearly the whole of them in the methods of physiological

---

[57] See Davis, 'Higher Education'.   [58] See Davis, 'Higher Education'.
[59] Royal Commission on Vivisection, 115–16, 144–6.
[60] Royal Commission on Vivisection, 190.

inquiry'.[61] William Rutherford had perfected his physiological skills in Berlin, Dresden, Prague, Vienna and Leipzig, where he also worked with Ludwig. He confessed that the 'tone of feeling' was rather higher among the 'English race', and that 'the amount of delicacy' in foreign hospitals was rather less. He also confessed that in England physiologists were 'more careful about repeating a painful experiment' than in Germany, and that the Germans went 'rather further' than he would have gone 'for the tuition of medical students'. Yet Rutherford had further to confess that he possessed this knowledge precisely because the German physiologists in Berlin and Leipzig had repeated painful experiments for him at his own request, 'as a person desirous of becoming a physiologist'. Hutton baited him with the suggestion that 'the Germans are as tender to pain generally as the English', but succumb to a greater 'zeal' in the pursuit of science. Rutherford's response is usefully demonstrative of the awkward position of English physiologists, caught among methodological appreciation, personal friendship, and home-grown moral boundaries:

I must decline to make any comparisons between the Germans and the English, because, although my physiological friends in Germany showed me some experiments which I do not think it necessary to repeat merely for the tuition of medical students, they showed me these experiments at my own request, and I thank them heartily for the gain to my knowledge. I really have had no personal experience of any unnecessary or reckless vivisection on any part of the Continent.[62]

Pushed a little further, Rutherford alluded to a difference in 'national temperament' to explain what may have looked like German indifference to suffering, but thought it 'a matter of opinion' whether 'men of that way of thinking might grow up in England'.[63] Nevertheless, he had previously opined freely on the difference in national temperament among German medical students compared with their English counterparts. German students, he said, 'are apparently a most tractable body in everything but politics. In class-rooms they are docile and passive, and are not given to knocking the dust off the floor, or other unwelcome demonstration of applause, such as an English professor is often troubled to control'. In short, a cold earnestness ran through German medical education, as much in the student body as in the professors. In a German lecture hall, 'no such sinful thought as that of perpetrating a practical joke during the lecture seems ever to enter their [the students'] heads; nay more, they attend their classes most assiduously,

[61] Royal Commission on Vivisection, 263.
[62] Royal Commission on Vivisection, 149, 156.
[63] Royal Commission on Vivisection, 156.

without the aid of cards or roll-call'.[64] But it was clear, to Rutherford at least, that the experience was essential for an English medical student:

the importance of knowing thoroughly those languages in which the best medical literature is contained, of becoming acquainted with those men who are the champions of medical science, of hearing the authors of some of the most important theories in medicine express and support them with their own lips, of being enabled to judge of the relative merits of various methods of treatment ... cannot be over-estimated.[65]

The younger generation of English and Scottish scientists insisted that German physiologists were ultimately humane, even if those men in Germany might have felt damned by faint praise. Acknowledging that occasionally they did go too far, their English pupils asserted that it did not follow that moral transgression inhered in the method itself. British physiologists felt perfectly assured in their assertion that experiences in a German laboratory as a kind of scientific finishing school had no diminishing effect on their status as English gentlemen, with all the moral sensibilities thereby implied.

Empty Rhetoric?

In the years following, German scientists would come to echo their English colleagues in claiming a greater and deeper form of humanity through their experimental practices while, at the same time, mocking the so-called refinement of English humanity and sensibility, which seemed to be dwarfed by English arrogance and aggression on the world stage. There was solidarity among professionals, to be sure, but each used clichés of the other's national character to claim distinction. Fundamentally, their arguments were the same. The problem, for English scientists, was that in denying that there was any danger of German brutality being adopted in English laboratories, they had tacitly acknowledged the existence of that brutality. It left them exposed. All of their high praise of German science was therefore undone by the testimony of one man.

Emanuel Klein, later known as Edward, was Slavonian, of Austrian descent. He trained in Vienna, and then worked in the laboratories of the German physiologist Ernst von Brücke (1819–92) and the Austrian pathologist Salomon Stricker (1834–98).[66] From 1871, Klein worked for the

---

[64] William Rutherford, 'The Chief Medical Schools of the Continent', *Edinburgh Medical Journal*, 11 (1865): 343. Rutherford's focus was mainly on Berlin, Vienna (which he referred to as 'German'), and Paris.

[65] Rutherford, 'Chief Medical Schools of the Continent', 347.

[66] Michael Worboys, 'Klein, Edward Emanuel (1844–1925)', in *Oxford Dictionary of National Biography* (Oxford: Oxford University Press, 2004), online edn, www

Brown Institute in London, under John Simon and John Burdon Sanderson. Here then, was a 'continental', Germanic in speech and training, in the midst of the English physiologists. Later, Klein claimed that he had been the victim of his poor English, not realizing the full ramifications of the questions posed to him. But for the antivivisectionists, and for Klein's English colleagues, his testimony before the Royal Commission seemed to provide all the ammunition necessary to make predictions about the moral future of Britain under the guidance of experimental scientists, who would doubtless succumb to the pernicious influence of their German methods. Moreover, he seemed to have pulled the wool over the eyes of his English employer, John Simon, who had already testified that the 'large practice of experiments' had 'produced no hardening effects at all with regard to [Klein's] sympathies with the lower animals'.[67]

Klein said he had 'No regard at all' for the sufferings of animals, and that he only used anaesthetics for convenience's sake, in order to hold the animal still. As a teacher, he used anaesthetics only because he considered the 'feelings and opinions of those people' who bore witness. Otherwise, he repeatedly attested his complete indifference to 'the sufferings of the animal', extending that principle to all the physiologists of Europe, and opining that there was no difference in feeling 'amongst the physiologists' in England. It was only the public in England which differed. In Europe, he said, 'the general public takes no view, does not claim to pronounce any criticism or any judgment about scientific teaching or physiology in general'.[68]

Klein horrified his colleagues, and afforded just the scandal desired by the antivivisectionist press.[69] He tried to undo the damage by amending his testimony after the fact, but the commission felt his amendments went beyond the bounds of acceptability. They were included in the appendix to the report. Klein tried to clarify that his indifference extended only to his own experiments, where the suffering was so minor as to be negligible. He also denied that he had any authority, as a foreigner, to pronounce on English physiologists, and claimed to be 'as much opposed as anyone in this country to unnecessary or unprofitable cruelty to animals'. He also added, in a bitter note, that the English public differed from the European chiefly in its disposition 'to take care of other people's consciences in

---

.oxforddnb.com/view/article/57359, accessed 1 February 2012. For Klein's involvement in the controversy, see Richards, 'Drawing the Life-Blood of Physiology', 44–5; Bruno Atalic and Stella Fatovic-Ferencic, 'Emanuel Edward Klein – The Father of British Microbiology and the Case of the Animal Vivisection Controversy of 1875', *Toxicologic Pathology*, 37 (2009): 708–13.

[67] Royal Commission on Vivisection, 74–5.
[68] Royal Commission on Vivisection, 183–5.
[69] See Richards, 'Drawing the Life-Blood of Physiology', 45.

matters they do not clearly understand'.[70] Despite the amendments, the damage was done. Vivisectionists were damned by association. The idea of the callous German scientist loomed large in the public imagination. It is difficult to measure the extent of the damage done by Klein in 1876, but it seemed to confirm that vivisection did require legislative regulation and that Germans ought not to be trusted. Back in Germany, the public would come to take an interest in the conscience of experimental science, even if those scientists would continue to emphasize that the public could not possibly understand.

Still, despite the cordial welcome given to German scientists at the IMC in 1881, the moral tone of men like Virchow at that event, and the lingering memory of Klein's testimony, meant that a coolness clouded the relationship of English and German scientists with respect to the defence of their practices. When John George Adami (1862–1926) translated Heidenhain's first pamphlet and offered it to the AAMR to be published, it was thought 'not ... advisable', with Brunton speculating that it had already been translated in America.[71] No such translation seems to have existed, and one need scarcely wonder why the AAMR Committee kept Heidenhain's work at arm's length. It is probable that such a clear demonstration of the association of English scientists and the Germans, to whom the former owed an enormous debt of gratitude in terms of formal instruction in method, was not desirable in an age where Germanness practically stood in for monstrousness in morals, especially as Heidenhain had himself previously condemned British morals in the form of imperialism. Adami had worked in Heidenhain's laboratory. A translation from this pen would have been too easily misinterpreted as another abandonment of English sensibilities.

This sense of distance was not replicated in the relationships of German and American medical scientists, which were only budding at this point. The highpoint of the American antivivisection movement would come only later, and the spectre of the brutal German scientist would linger. Just as the bright young things of England had completed their training in European laboratories of note, so too did American medical researchers blood themselves abroad. Henry Pickering Bowditch, about whom much more will be said in the following chapter, completed his American education at Harvard, either side of the Civil War (in which he served as Major). Armed with his medical degree, Bowditch went first to study with Claude Bernard, the father of physiology, in Paris, but ultimately found his way to Germany. He studied first at Bonn with Wilhelm Kühne and Max Schultze and then went on

---

[70] Royal Commission on Vivisection, 183–5, 328.   [71] AAMR Minutes, 44.

to Leipzig and the laboratory of Ludwig. Ludwig's physiological programme would form the basis of Bowditch's own at Harvard. Indeed, it
was Bowditch who broadcast Ludwig's celebrated laboratory-complex
design to the world, first in the *Boston Medical and Surgical Journal* and
afterwards in *Nature*.[72] Bowditch was in Germany until 1871, prior to
any antivivisection controversy there, and therefore took back to
Harvard an idealized view of German methods, German technology
and the German ethos of physiological research. He was appointed
Assistant Professor of Physiology in 1871 and, under the presidentship
of Charles Eliot (1834–1926) (who would come to be a great ally of
American medical research), essentially founded the discipline of physiology in America on German lines.

Bowditch's experience was not untypical. The leading lights in American
medical research from the 1870s all had spells in Europe. W. W. Keen
(1837–1932) spent time in Paris and Berlin; William H. Welch (1850–
1934) was, like Bowditch, inspired by Ludwig's laboratory in Leipzig,
having spent time working with Julius Cohnheim (1839–84) and Virchow,
and inaugurated his Bellevue Medical College laboratory on Ludwig's lines
in 1877, before opening a more important venture on similar lines at the new
Johns Hopkins Hospital and Medical School in 1884. These would be some
of the giants of the development and institutionalization of American medical research, which had its Germanness built in. To this were added
a number of German emigrés, such as Jacques Loeb (1859–1924) at
Chicago. They built physiological laboratories and expanded programmes
of physiological research, untrammelled by controversy.

When the controversy came, later, it contained barbs against German
brutality and its institutionalization in American laboratories, though not
to the extent that Germanness worried the older English medical establishment. Albert Leffingwell (1845–1916), an important antivivisectionist
because of his claim to medical credentials (even though most physiologists recognized him as a crank), wrote a pamphlet in 1900 with the title
'Is Science Advanced by Deceit'.[73] In it, he denounced Goltz for cutting
off the breasts of a dog. The charge rankled. Jacques Loeb and Bowditch
discussed it, berating Leffingwell's misunderstanding of Goltz's German
and calling him a liar. Loeb called upon Bowditch to do something about
this deceit, to rally with those who had 'taken up the fight'.[74] Bowditch

---

[72] H. P. Bowditch, 'The Physiological Laboratory at Leipzig', *Nature*, 3 (1870): 142–3.

[73] Albert Leffingwell, *Is Science Advanced by Deceit? A Question and a Criticism* (Providence,
RI: American Humane Association, 1900).

[74] Loeb to Bowditch, 11 December 1900, and Loeb to Bowditch, 23 February 1901, H MS
c 40, Folder 306, Box 26, Walter B. Cannon Archive, Countway Library of Medicine,
Boston (WBCA).

would himself equivocate on the matter of German moral fibre, remarking on one occasion that there was 'no doubt . . . that the French and Germans are less careful than the Anglo-Saxons are in regard to the sufferings of animals', but the observation did not stand in the way of his leadership on behalf of experimental medicine in America.[75] It would not be a fight for German methods so much as it was a defence of American humanity, and it is to that fight that we now turn.

[75] Transcript of hearing at Boston State House on bill relating to vivisection, 12 March 1896, H MS c 40, Folder 292, Box 24, WBCA, 40.

3   Of Laboratories and Legislatures

The Great Educator

'A cat has the same senses possessed by man in a more acute form.' So ran the cursive chalk writing on the blackboard of the 'Great Educator', Satanus Inferno, a devil in morning suit and top hat, whose chief object was to teach 'the children and youth in our American schools' how to cut off the heads of live cats (Figure 3.1). The schoolchildren, assembled in front of the board in well-to-do attire, brandish cats by the neck and tail, armed with sharp knives. One enterprising boy has the head of a cat on his knife – a keener, clearly – having decapitated it before the teacher had dispatched his own. The image appeared in the supplement to the June 1897 issue of *Our Dumb Animals*, which claimed to speak on behalf of the Massachusetts Society for the Prevention of Cruelty to Animals (MSPCA), the American Humane Education Society, and the American Bands of Mercy. The previous year, the MSPCA had tried to bring into law an Act to prevent painful experimentation on animals in all educational institutions in Massachusetts, unless authorized by the State Board of Health and attended by a representative of the MSPCA. The Bill was watered down in successive versions, and ultimately dismissed. Whatever rhetorical claims to moderation the Bill's sponsors may have claimed, the medical profession understood them to be depicting scientists as immoral, cruel and beastly. Images such as this, in the Society's official organ, did little to dispel the thought that the antivivisectionists' principal objection was that scientists were corrupting the youth. It drew the ire of the medical-scientific establishment.

Foundations

For Henry Pickering Bowditch, physiological research and the education of students in physiology was 'humanity in its highest state'. That, at any rate, was what he wrote to the Massachusetts Society for the Prevention of

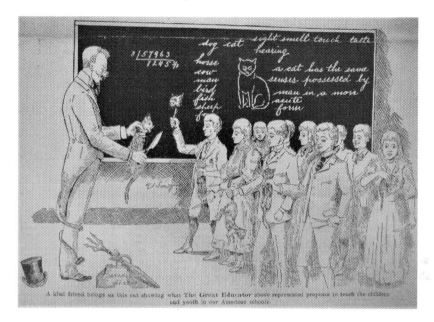

Figure 3.1 'The Great Educator', *Our Dumb Animals*, supplement to June 1897.

Cruelty to Animals to notify them that he was withdrawing his support and annual contribution of $5. His 'confidence in the wisdom' of the Society's administration had been 'shaken' by its antagonism to this 'humanity', which it had 'allowed itself to be drawn into' while interfering with the State's education policy.[1] While neither Bowditch's subscription form nor his appended letter are dated, they are likely from around 1896, coincident with the aforementioned Bill. Bowditch spoke at three hearings pertaining to the Bill at Boston State House in the early months of 1896.[2] In the same year, a restrictive Bill was also entered in the US Senate. By that point, Bowditch had already been involved in rallying the scientific defence of animal experimentation for a decade. The MSPCA had been involved in an Act of 1894 that prohibited vivisection in public schools, and in early 1896, the Massachusetts Medical Society (MMS) wrote formally to tell the MSPCA to back off. Bowditch was copied in on the correspondence, which stated that vivisection was not 'practised in this State in an unnecessary or

---

[1] Subscription letter for the MSPCA with appended letter in Bowditch's hand, undated. H MS c 40, Folder 291, Box 24, WBCA.

[2] Transcript of hearing at Boston State House on bill relating to vivisection, H MS c 40, Folder 292, Box 24, WBCA.

cruel manner'; that 'the existing statutes furnish sufficient security against cruelty in vivisection', and that 'experience has shown it to be very undesirable to impose restrictions of any kind upon the advancement of medical science by the researches of properly qualified persons'. Thus, they reported that it was 'inexpedient to legislate upon this subject'.[3] This was a remarkably coherent stance, though it did not immediately stay the action of the MSPCA and its president, George Angell (1823–1909). Still, it is representative of a well-thought-out principle. From where did it spring?

For about fifteen years, work at Bowditch's German-style laboratory at Harvard had progressed without hindrance. The biological laboratory at Johns Hopkins University in Baltimore had only opened in 1876. A decade or so later, the head of that laboratory, H. Newell Martin (1848–96), together with Silas Weir Mitchell (1829–1914) of the University of Pennsylvania, and Bowditch at Harvard, helped found the American Physiological Society. H. Newell Martin was particularly disposed to be part of such an organization. He called for physiologists to 'combine' in 1885 in his response to a slanderous attack on his work and character in Frances Power Cobbe's journal *The Zoophilist*. He asked if it were not 'our duty to protect the general public from being led astray by falsehood', in order to continue unhindered with research into the 'conditions of health, and the methods of preventing and curing disease in man and the lower animals'. 'Truth', he averred, 'cannot hurt' and the 'world made better as well as happier, through our researches'. Laboratory experimentation in America was, belatedly, on the map.[4] Still, as Jutta Schickore has observed, it was hardly a mainstream medical activity. According to one estimate, in 1883 vivisection-based experiments only took place in five American cities.[5] If antivivisection was alive in America before the mid 1880s, it had very little to aim at. Slowly, that changed, and from the outset, American antivivisectionists targeted both State and Federal legislation as the most likely way to generate support and to secure change. Medical scientists, and Bowditch chief among them, found themselves having to work beyond the laboratory, making a case for laboratory work in the legislature.

William H. Welch soon rose to prominence at Johns Hopkins, and with him a model of scientific practice and of the scientific self was formed and subsequently bequeathed to many of the next generation's most

---

[3] F. W. Goss to Bowditch, 24 February 1896. H MS c 40, Folder 289, Box 24, WBCA.

[4] For context, W. Bruce Fye, *The Development of American Physiology: Scientific Medicine in the Nineteenth Century* (Baltimore: Johns Hopkins University Press, 1987); H. Newell Martin, *A Correction of Certain Statements in the 'Zoophilist', also A Castigation and an Appeal* [pamphlet] (Baltimore, 1885), 10.

[5] Schickore, *About Method*, 145. Baltimore, Boston, New York, Philadelphia, Easton, Pa.

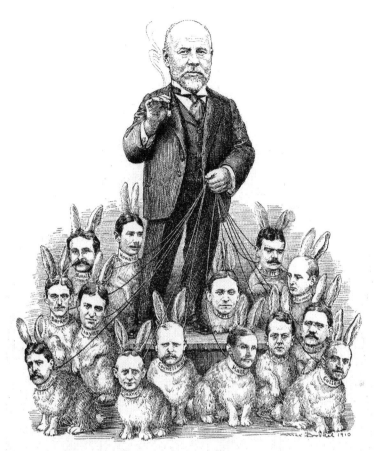

Some Welch rabbits

Figure 3.2 Max Broedel, 'Some Welch Rabbits', 1910. Wellcome Library, London. Attribution 4.0 International (CC BY 4.0).

influential experimenters (Figure 3.2). With wry wit, he was depicted by Max Broedel (1870–1941) in 1910 holding the leashes of the great and good of the American medical-scientific community, whom he had trained, represented as so many laboratory rabbits. Together with Bowditch, Welch framed the American ethos of medical research, its 'epistemic virtue', to borrow a phrase from Lorraine Daston and Peter

Galison, and its essential moral justification.[6] Perhaps 'justification' is too negative. Welch and Bowditch did not apologize for their vivisection activities. Rather, they posited them as a moral imperative. In 1886, Welch explicitly argued the case for the 'humanity' of medical science, noting that bacteriological experimentation had led to new knowledge that would prevent disease. It was 'destined' to do good.[7] Only a few years later, Bowditch wrote of the immense value of immunological research, which had replaced 'despair' with 'a feeling of well grounded hope' among physicians, and which had removed the 'burden of terror and distress' from bedside witnesses. It was a 'boon', purchased cheaply 'by the lives of some thousands of guinea pigs'.[8] Who could, with reason, declare otherwise? This kind of rhetoric was designed to show that experimental medicine had not abandoned tender feelings for the sake of the pursuit of knowledge. On the contrary, it entwined humanity with reason and pointed to the irrationality and unbounded sentimentality of the other side.

The American medical establishment had the benefit of time to prepare. They knew, as their own research programmes expanded, that it was but a matter of time before antivivisection found a footing somewhere. In early 1887, the Medical Society of the State of New York had elected Bowditch to its Committee on Experimental Medicine and resolved to prepare to arrest and confront the antivivisection movement. John C. Dalton (1825–89), the Secretary to the Society, wrote to Bowditch that 'we are extending our ramifications, to be ready for future contests with the antivivisection hysterics'.[9]

Dalton had been America's first Professor of Physiology, appointed in 1851 in Buffalo after a year studying with Claude Bernard in Paris. Afterwards, he had moved to New York and had been perhaps the first American physiologist to warn against antivivisection and to justify the experimental method in humane terms. He wrote the first American text book on human physiology in 1859, following it with a number of monographs designed specifically to uphold physiology's methods in the face of charges of inhumanity. Of these, his *Experimentation on Animals, as a Means of Knowledge in Physiology* (1875) and *Experimental Method in Medical Science* (1882), as well as an essay in the *Bulletin of the New York Academy of Medicine* on 'Vivisection: What It Is, and What It Has Accomplished' (1867) set the tone, the message and framed the argument

---

[6] Daston and Galison, *Objectivity*.

[7] William H. Welch, 'On Some of the Humane Aspects of Medical Science', *Papers and Addresses* (Baltimore: Johns Hopkins University Press, 1920), 3:4.

[8] Henry Pickering Bowditch, 'The Advancement of Medicine by Research', *Science*, 4 (1896): 99.

[9] Dalton to Bowditch, 31 January 1887, H MS c 40, Folder 2897, Box 24, WBCA.

that would dominate political wrangling over vivisection in America up to the First World War. Dalton was ahead of his time, in touch with arguments that were burgeoning in England, and he was motivated to inform his colleagues. In his 1875 book he particularly took issue with the question of humanity and inhumanity. 'The charge of inhumanity, as brought against the practice of experimentation on animals', he wrote, 'seems to ignore in great measure the motive and object of such investigations'. Scientists could not be cruel because their object was 'solely the acquisition of a kind of knowledge which has been shown to be inferior to none in its importance for the welfare of mankind'.[10] Dalton died before seeing any real threat to American physiology, but he had prepared the ground, locking horns with the founder of the American Society for the Prevention of Cruelty to Animals (founded 1866), Henry Bergh (1813–88). Bergh had quickly turned his sights on medical experimentation, but made little headway. It was he who introduced a Bill in the New York State Legislature in 1880 designed to prohibit vivisection, which was a resolute failure.

In response the Medical Society of the State of New York formed a Committee on Experimental Medicine in 1881, 'charged with the duty' of preventing 'harmful interference' in experimental work. This was announced in a circular sent to members of the American Society for the Prevention of Cruelty to Animals, noting the 'desire' of experimenters to 'prevent every form of unnecessary suffering' and of the virtues of the 'careful use of the lower animals for the benefit of humanity and of the brute creation'.[11] The prohibitory Bill was reintroduced in 1881, but again failed to progress. A relative calm then ensued. In the interim, Dalton prepared Bowditch, telling him that while there was no 'indication of immediate bother', one could never rest easily with 'such self righteous busy bodies as Bergh and his imitators'. He told Bowditch that the 'policy' should be 'to pay no public attention to them until they attempt something real in the way of legislation, but to be prepared beforehand so that we can act then with unanimity and promptness'. Dalton was convinced that a policy of non-engagement in public would succeed, waiting instead until 'they attack us openly in the legislature', where 'we can beat them every time'. He warned Bowditch that members of the legislature 'will always be guided, as a whole, by their family doctors, or the best ones in their vicinity',

[10] 'John C. Dalton, Jr. (1825–1889) Experimental Physiologist', *Journal of the American Medical Association*, 203 (1968): 155–6.
[11] Circular letter of the Medical Society of the State of New York to the Officers and Members of the American Society for the Prevention of Cruelty to Animals, H MS c 40, Folder 295, Box 24, WBCA.

so such men had 'to be notified early enough beforehand, to know what the danger is that threatens'.[12] Such would be the policy, up until 1908.

Bowditch also prepared himself, being physically present at the meeting of the Physiological Society during the IMC in 1881 where the coordinated defence of experiment began in England. He capitalized on these early preparations and warning shots, sending a circular letter in 1895 to experts across the country looking for potential committee members and specialists to speak and write in favour of vivisection. Replies came in the affirmative from throughout the Midwest and the East Coast, from Chicago and Cincinnati, from Boston, Baltimore and Yale. Warren P. Lombard (1855–1939), Professor of Physiology and Histology at the University of Michigan had trained under Bowditch and, following his lead, had gone to Germany to hone his expertise, spending two years under Ludwig at Leipzig. He answered Bowditch's call positively, endorsing 'the plan of arming during peace in order to prevent war', but urged Bowditch to 'keep the fact as quiet as may be until the time comes to strike ... without an appeal to the public'. After all, 'the sensationalist has the advantage every time'.[13] The advice, which would characterize the course of the American defence over a generation, was clearly well heeded.

If Bowditch had been alerted to the potential of trouble by Dalton, he was confirmed in it by indirect communication with Michael Foster in England. The year after Dalton's death, Clifton Hodge (1859–1949), a newly appointed Professor of Physiology at Clark University (who had trained at Hopkins), was the recipient of Foster's letter, but he forwarded it to Bowditch. It affords candid insight into Foster's feelings on the legislative restrictions on experimental work that arose after the Act of 1876. Foster is full of bile and regret that more was not done to prevent the passage of the Bill. He regretted the lost time and the lost opportunities, and warned Hodge that any similar legislation in America would 'worry' science – that is, it would strangle and suffocate it. The legislation had passed in England because upper-middle-class 'doctrinaires' had had the 'time and funds for public agitation, while men of science and doctors had something else to do and hated agitation'. They had fallen sleepily into legislative regulation out of distaste for public bickering and because they had failed to see the severity of the threat. Foster could not have been clearer about his regrets in this regard, written in the form of a call to arms among American scientists:

But if the time were to come over again, I should fight tooth and nail against any act at all, on the ground that all such *legislative restrictions are unnecessary*, – that

---

[12] Dalton to Bowditch, June 29 [no year, but 1889 or before], H MS c 40, Folder 290, Box 24, WBCA.
[13] Lombard to Bowditch, 12 December 1895, H MS c 40, Folder 288, Box 24, WBCA.

instances of cruelty, that is of heedless causing of pain on the part of physiologists, are to say the least, rare, and that public opinion aided by the ordinary law is quite sufficient to cope with such cases.... And much as I hate public agitation, I should throw myself with all the energy I possess into agitating against such measures sacrificing my little portion of present science for the sake of science to come. My advice to you is, accept no compromise whatever, refuse to admit for a moment the need of such a law, and fight against it everywhere, in the newspapers and on the platform, and if the situation demands it, even imitate your opponents and refuse a political vote against it. I don't think I can say anything stronger than this last. To repeal a law is a very different thing from opposing the making of one. I scarcely think that I shall live to see the repeal of our Act, but if the chance of success ever offers itself I trust I should be ready to carry out for ourselves the advice which I am now giving you.[14]

Hodge, at a junior stage of his career, doubtless thought this incendiary letter merited attention and authority beyond what he could muster by himself, though he did quote it in an article published in the autumn of 1896.[15] He forecast that antivivisection would foster its own demise, through its dubious 'methods of agitation'. But by handing the letter to Bowditch, the leading figure in American physiology and already primed for defence by association with Dalton, he provided him with the spirit, motivation and style of the American defence of experimental medicine. Foster's advice regarding the press, the platform and the legislature, was followed to the letter over the following generation, and Bowditch would be the first of many – Harold Ernst (1856–1922), Walter Cannon (1871–1945), Simon Flexner (1863–1946), Frederick Schiller Lee (1859–1939) – who would, as Foster thought he might have done, sacrifice their own time as scientists to ensure that those who followed would not have to. The advice of the MMS to the MSPCA seems as if lifted directly from Foster's guidance. Its spirit would see Bowditch and his colleagues compelled away from the laboratory and into the legislature and its principal mode, rhetoric.

Honing the Argument

As in Germany, the roots of antivivisectionism in America are traceable to England. Bergh inspired Caroline Earl White (1833–1916), founder of the Pennsylvania Society for the Prevention of Cruelty to Animals in 1867 and, in 1883, of the American Anti-Vivisection Society. In the latter activity she

[14] An excerpt of the letter was later entered as part of William Welch's remonstrance against an antivivisectionist Bill in the U.S. Senate to restrict vivisection in the District of Columbia, in 1900. 98–9.
[15] C. F. Hodge, *The Vivisection Question*, reprinted from *Appleton's Popular Science Monthly*, September and October, 1896, 26.

'fell under the personal spell' of Frances Power Cobbe.[16] A slew of other local societies followed. As per Susan Lederer's observation on the movement, it was powered by women, who comprised the bulk of subscribers to these societies and to their publications.[17] Yet if the antivivisectionists looked to England for their arguments and tactics, so did the scientists.

Bowditch had been collecting literature produced by the English antivivisection movement since 1875.[18] He knew its rhetoric and the likelihood that it would be reproduced in America. As home-grown organizations – the American Humane Association, the New England Anti-vivisection Society, the Illinois Anti-vivisection Society, the MSPCA – began to produce their own antivivisection material, Bowditch scrupulously collected all of that too.[19] The appearance, in 1896, in the US Senate of Bill 1552, which aimed to curb the freedom with which medical scientists could employ animals for experimental purposes in the District of Columbia, was perhaps the first real cause for alarm: a signal moment that the general increase in antivivisection agitation, especially in New York and Massachusetts, might strike a victory in the District of Columbia, at some distance from the front lines. The Senator responsible for championing it was an extra cause for alarm. Jacob Harold Gallinger (1837–1918) had, prior to his political career, long served as a practising physician, having obtained a medical degree from Cincinnati in 1858. Medical scientists were always more alarmed by threats to their profession that came from within, especially from members whose active knowledge of more recent advances in medical training (and especially of the value of physiology) were entirely missing. Gallinger fit the bill as a tricky opponent. C. W. Dabney (1855–1945), the Assistant Secretary of the US Department of Agriculture, for example, was alarmed, sending a circular letter warning of the disastrous effect of any successful legislation on the work of the Bureau of Animal Industry of the Department of Agriculture, which was 'doing work of the highest grade and of the greatest value to humanity', framed as the protection of agricultural animals that were the source of nourishment for the nation. He called for 'everyone interested in these scientific investigations' to write 'at once to both of the Senators from

---

[16] Susan Lederer, 'The Controversy over Animal Experimentation in America, 1880–1914', in *Vivisection in Historical Perspective*, ed. Nicolaas Rupke (London: Croom Helm, 1987), 238.

[17] Lederer, 'Controversy', 239. See also Craig Buettinger, 'Women and Antivivisection in Late Nineteenth-Century America', *Journal of Social History*, 30 (1997): 857–72.

[18] H MS c 40, Folder 298, Box 25, WBCA.

[19] H MS c 40, Folder 299, Box 25, WBCA; H MS c 40, Folder 300, Box 25, WBCA; H MS c 40, Folder 301, Box 25, WBCA; H MS c 40, Folder 302, Box 25, WBCA; H MS c 40, Folder 303, Box 25, WBCA.

his State and to the Representative from his district expressing disapproval'.[20]

Compliance with this request was thoroughgoing. Among Bowditch's papers, filed with those of Walter Cannon in Boston, is a typed memorandum written under the auspices of the National Academy of Sciences, with pencil annotations in Bowditch's hand. Bowditch had been elected to the Academy in 1887, and by 1896 he was helping to steer its official policy with respect to animal experimentation. Bowditch's tone was stark. The memo reads: 'The physiologist, no less than the physicist and the chemist, can expect advancement of his science only as the result of carefully planned laboratory work.' Here Bowditch inserted: 'If this work is interfered with medical science will continue to advance, as heretofore by means of experiment, for no legislation can affect the position of physiology as an experimental science; but there will be this important difference, that the experimenters will be medical practitioners & the victims human beings.'

Bowditch's threat was palpable, tapping into the oft-stated fear of antivivisectionists that vivisection was the gateway to human abuses, contorting that fear to make vivisection the bulwark against such abuses. The threat was also singular. While it established the ardour with which American medical scientists would commit themselves to the cause, it was not politically wise to draw attention to the very spectre that underwrote so much antivivisectionist rhetoric. While the memorandum made clear that the 'men engaged in this work are activated by motives no less humane than those which guide the person who desire to restrict their action', Bowditch's amendment hinted at a callousness contained only by practicality, and of a general misgiving about American medical practice.[21] The memorandum would be compiled, together with similar resolutions from the American Medical Association, the Association of American Medical Colleges, the Association of American Physicians, the Medical Society of the District of Columbia, the Joint Commission of the Scientific Societies, the American Academy of Medicine, the Biological Society of Washington, the Washington Chemical Society, the Entomological Society of Washington and the Philosophical Society of Washington, and issued as a pamphlet under the title *Defence of Vivisection*.[22] William Patten (1861–1932), Professor of Zoology and General Biology at Dartmouth, wrote to Gallinger under the auspices of the American Society of Naturalists and the American Society of

---

[20] Chas. W. Dabney, Circular No. 4, H MS c 40, Folder 294, Box 24, WBCA.

[21] No date, no title, memorandum of the National Academy of Sciences to the Members of Congress, H MS c 40, Folder 289, Box 24, WBCA.

[22] *Defence of Vivisection*, H MS c 40, Folder 295, Box 24, WBCA.

Embryologists to point out that vivisectors – 'educated, humane, and intelligent men' – would employ their own 'sense of humanity and self protection', which could be relied upon to suppress abuses.[23] At the heart of American democracy, the establishment were ranged in defiant opposition to antivivisection measures from the start.

Against such a line-up, the Bill quickly went away, only to be reintroduced in subsequent years (Bills 1063 and 34). This would be the pattern in DC and in states with major areas of animal research – New York, Boston, Baltimore, Chicago – placing a new burden on medical scientists to become part-time professional remonstrants against antivivisectionist legislation. The organization of the scientists improved accordingly. Bowditch took Gallinger directly to task in private correspondence, accusing him of 'a too great readiness to trust the extravagant statements of men and women whose zeal has outrun their discretion'.[24] By reply, Gallinger pooh-poohed the whole notion of 'eminence' as anything to go by, and implied that if trust in antivivisectionist cant was the Scylla to be avoided, then 'giving implicit confidence to the statements of scientific vivisectors regarding vivisection' was the Charybdis.[25] It was this lack of implicit trust or respect that made Gallinger seem so dangerous. Bowditch implored Gallinger to become personally informed about laboratory procedures – Bowditch offered him a standing invitation to visit his laboratory – so that he 'would be convinced that physiologists are guided by motives no less humane and far more intelligent than those which actuate the men and women who denounce them as "cowardly criminals"'. He closed by begging Gallinger to 'believe that physiologists are not necessarily inhumane because, in seeking the good of the human race, they follow Nature's example in sacrificing the lower to the higher forms of life'.[26] Gallinger's views notwithstanding, a broad respect for eminence, and an implicit trust and confidence in the humanity of medical science would, ultimately, count for everything in the defence of experimental medicine. In early 1898, William H. Welch, then acting as President of the Congress of American Physicians and Surgeons, formed a committee of experts to oppose Bill 1063, asking Bowditch to serve. He also wrote to two prominent physicians in each state to beg them to write personal letters of opposition, and to enjoin them to persuade others to do the same.[27] The network was easily mobilized.

---

[23] Patten to Gallinger (copy of letter dated 25 January 1896), H MS c 40, Folder 289, Box 24, WBCA.

[24] Bowditch to Gallinger, 27 May 1897, H MS c 40, Folder 290, Box 24, WBCA.

[25] Gallinger to Bowditch, 3 June 1897, H MS c 40, Folder 290, Box 24, WBCA.

[26] Bowditch to Gallinger, 12 June 1897, H MS c 40, Folder 290, Box 24, WBCA.

[27] Welch to Bowditch, 5 January 1898, H MS c 40, Folder 290, Box 24, WBCA. For context, Patricia Peck Gossel, 'William Henry Welch and the Antivivisection Legislation

As mentioned above, the first Bill in DC happened in the same year as the first antivivisectionist Bill in Massachusetts, and Bowditch organized his colleagues and allies accordingly. Bowditch himself played a major role, pointing to the 'misguided benevolence' of antivivisection activism. It was, he said, a movement that appealed 'to some of our noblest feelings, to the sentiment that bids us be merciful as we would obtain mercy', its advocates being largely of a 'benevolent ... disposition and conscientious in their attitude'. But they were lacking in 'common sense', which could lead to 'folly, which is but the handmaiden of crime'.[28] At the third hearing, in April 1896, Bowditch and his peers presented the kind of animal research being undertaken in Massachusetts laboratories, with an emphasis on painlessness and on the use of anaesthesia, as well as on the 'humane' killing of animals prior to regaining consciousness. Emphasis was also placed, by Hodge, on dangers of the 'easily convinced woman', whose sentiments were too easily stirred by lies, misdirection and misrepresentation.[29] These were contrasted, by Theobald Smith (1859–1934), with the experimentalists' vision of the progress of civilization and the need for continued animal experimentation in order to keep up with 'new conditions'.[30] Yet the emotional core of the remonstrance lay in the words of the Harvard President, Charles W. Eliot, who pointed out the thousands of 'humane young men' who, over two decades, had borne witness to the work of the physiological laboratory at Harvard and had gone on to become 'much trusted men'. That the MSPCA was sponsoring the legislation was said by Eliot to strike a chord with the public that these men were 'cruel to animals', pursued a 'cruel vocation', which would, if true, be 'criminal'. Eliot vouchsafed for 'these gentlemen' that they were the 'most humane and truly merciful men in the whole community'. Here was 'a calm, slow-burning, but steady enthusiasm for the prevention and cure' of diseases. Eliot claimed that a 'man's daily occupation, followed for years, tells in his face' and he submitted that the men who had remonstrated with the committee formed to consider the Bill wore faces that 'tell that they are humane, merciful, clear-seeing men, devoted for life to the most humane occupation now existing in the world'.[31] Trust, so the argument went, was etched into the very visage of

---

in the District of Columbia, 1896–1900', *Journal of the History of Medicine and Allied Sciences*, 40 (1985): 397–419.

[28] Transcript of hearing at Boston State House on bill relating to vivisection, 12 March 1896, H MS c 40, Folder 292, Box 24, WBCA, 19–20.

[29] Transcript of hearing at Boston State House on bill providing for inspection of vivisection experiments, 2 April 1896, H MS c 40, Folder 293, Box 24, WCBA, 12.

[30] Transcript of hearing at Boston State House on bill providing for inspection of vivisection experiments, 2 April 1896, H MS c 40, Folder 293, Box 24, WCBA, 20.

[31] Transcript of hearing at Boston State House on bill providing for inspection of vivisection experiments, 2 April 1896, H MS c 40, Folder 293, Box 24, WCBA, 16–17.

the physiologist. To legislate along the lines of mistrust was an insult. To impugn their humanity was to misunderstand what humanity was.

The hearing for the 1899 DC Bill took place in February 1900, with Gallinger aided and abetted by Albert Leffingwell. Opposed to them were an extraordinary array of the medical establishment's great and good, introduced by William Williams Keen (1837–1932), the pioneering brain surgeon, including, by correspondence, such luminaries at Lord Lister, Thomas Lauder Brunton and Michael Foster from England. In person speakers included three of the Baltimore big four, the celebrated physician and transatlantic defender of the profession, William Osler; the pioneering gynaecologist, Howard Kelly (1858–1943); and Johns Hopkins Medical School's founding professor, William H. Welch. Bowditch was there, of course, as was H. A. Hare (1862–1931) of Jefferson Medical College. Important medical figures in government departments showed up, including the Surgeon General of the US Army, George M. Sternberg (1838–1915), and D. E. Salmon (1850–1914), the Chief of the Bureau of the Animal Industry in the Department of Agriculture (and who gave his name to salmonella). Another important figure was Mary Putnam Jacobi (1842–1906), whose status as a leading figure in the treatment of disease was enhanced, in this case, by her being a woman. In a controversy often couched heavily in terms of gendered emotion – antivivisection was dubbed an instance of misplaced sentiment, reaching hysterical levels – a woman's voice of reason from within the ranks of medical expertise was considered enormously valuable.[32]

The coordination of the defence was no accident, but the result of a well-connected and sharply organized correspondence network that had, through the experience of Bowditch and others, thoroughly rehearsed the arguments in favour of animal experimentation. Those arguments included summaries of the measurable impact of vivisection in terms of the increase of medical knowledge and the reduction of both human and animal suffering. But it was the moral demeanour of the assembled scientists – the affective mode of delivery of these arguments – that was key. Not only were they to be trusted for their expertise, but because such expertise could only have been won by those with hearts in the best of condition. Keen set the tone, leading off the remonstrances. Not only was vivisection right, but it was a 'duty to perform it'. Comparing the medical establishment to their opponents he pointed out that they also were 'stirred ... by emotions – emotions of pity,

---

[32] For one interpretation of the report of the hearing, see Thomas A. Woolsey and Robert E. Burke, 'The Playwright, the Practitioner, the Politician, the President, and the Pathologist: A Guide to the 1900 Senate Document Titled "Vivisection"', *Perspectives in Biology and Medicine*, 30 (1987): 235–58.

emotions of sympathy, and emotions of love – not only for our fellow men, but also for animals. We love them just as well, but we love them, as we think, more wisely'.[33] He went on that it was his 'duty', his 'highest duty', to 'see whether on animals some other method of operating will not enable' him to 'save life'.[34] Keen recounted a story of being refused a dog from the pound of the Women's Branch of the Pennsylvania Society for the Prevention of Cruelty to Animals, from which to extract a nerve with which to save an injured man from suffering. The refusal, he said, 'shows the profound cruelty of our opponents'.[35]

This was to be the classic reversal: to reflect the charge of cruelty back upon those who made just that accusation of medical scientists. Taken as a whole, the rhetorical position reframed virtuous emotion and moral disposition in terms of the expertise and practice of experimenters, not simply denying humane intentions to antivivisectionists (who were assumed to be honestly motivated for the most part), but denying them the capacity of humanity because they lacked both experience and expertise in the things they criticized. Bowditch doubled down on the argument, repeating his exact sentiments from 1896 in Massachusetts about 'misguided benevolence' and suggesting that the success of the antivivisection movement would plunge medical science 'into a darkness worse than medieval'.[36] And Mary Putnam Jacobi pointed out the absurdity of a 'dangerously demagogic inversion of the proper relation of knowledge and ignorance' if the layperson were appointed to oversea and adjudge the practices of 'scientific men'. The Government of the USA, she said, was 'radically, necessarily, intrinsically unfit' to 'meddle' with such work.[37] Not letting the opportunity slip, in a characteristic remark Putnam Jacobi said that the 'readiness on the part of women to plunge into active meddling with what they know nothing about, is one of the consequences of the privation of political rights, which forcibly expresses their instincts for public activities'. In her opinion, political enfranchisement would direct them to more 'legitimate' activities and they would 'cease these excited crusades on matters about which only very few can, or care to, know'.[38]

---

[33] US Congress, 56th sess. (1899–1900), Senate, 'Vivisection. Hearing before the Senate Committee on the District of Columbia, February 21, 1900, on the Bill (S. 34) for the further prevention of cruelty to animals in the District of Columbia' (Washington, DC: Government Printing Office, 1900), 24.

[34] US Congress, 'Vivisection', 27.   [35] US Congress, 'Vivisection', 28.

[36] US Congress, 'Vivisection', 55–6.   [37] US Congress, 'Vivisection', 59–60.

[38] US Congress, 'Vivisection', 60. For context, Carla Bittel, 'Science, Suffrage, and Experimentation: Mary Putnam Jacobi and the Controversy over Vivisection in Late Nineteenth-Century America', *Bulletin of the History of Medicine*, 79 (2005): 664–94; Regina Markell Morantz, 'Feminism, Professionalism, and Germs: The Thought of Mary Putnam Jacobi and Elizabeth Blackwell', *American Quarterly*, 34 (1982): 459–78.

William Osler called the American Humane Association, which had busied itself in advertising experimental abuses within inexpert medical research, 'disgraceful', and denounced the opponents of vivisection who came from within the medical profession as his 'bitterest enemies': 'With reference to men who train with these enemies of the profession I say this, that I scorn them from my heart. They may know that they have the scorn of a man who has the respect of his fellow-members in the profession to which I belong'. It was an extraordinary outburst, in defence of the honour of the medical establishment, of men 'who daily give up their lives for their fellows.' Osler's word carried great weight. His 'blood ... surged in [his] veins' hearing the medical profession calumniated in a public forum.[39] It was rare public display of anger among the defenders of medical research, but it was consciously grounded in a context of humanity, of the focus of the profession on the suffering of the other.

In practical terms, the honing of the argument also drew heavily on the experience of English and Scottish scientists who had felt their own practice to have been disturbed by the law of 1876. Whatever the actual circumstances of the situation in England, where the AAMR on the whole successfully navigated the law to the great benefit of medical researchers, there was no shortage of testimony from eminent men, in the form of letters solicited by men like Keen, pertaining to the great hardships and restrictions occasioned by the law. The specific machinery of the medical negotiation of the Act remained completely invisible in public discourse outside of England (indeed, it was practically invisible in England), such that English medical researchers presented a picture of being hampered in the extreme by the regulative legislation. Lister, for example, dwelt on his early and privately conducted experiments on frogs – experiments conducted in his own house – which were the gateway to a life of science and esteemed discovery, to the great benefit of humanity. Such experiments, he said, would have been denied under the 1876 Act, and who knew how many advances were at that moment being retarded by the law.[40] In a context that was constructed to portray the honourable nature of the vast majority of men working in the field, such words hit home. The fame of the names in question only gave the words greater bearing.

Organization Fatigue

There was an antivivisection Bill in Massachusetts in 1900, for which Bowditch led the remonstrants. Organization of the defence was directed by Harold C. Ernst (1856–1922). Ernst was a Harvard bacteriologist who,

[39] US Congress, 'Vivisection', 65.   [40] US Congress, 'Vivisection', 96–7.

under Bowditch's direction, had confirmed Koch's work on tuberculosis in the early 1880s, afterwards going to Berlin to work directly with Koch. According to Ernst's biography, his time with Koch made him a 'proselytizer of European bacteriology to the American medical profession'.[41] He was one of the Harvard men responsible for diphtheria antitoxin research and antitoxin production, but was superseded by Theobald Smith (to whom Eliot referred as the peerless expert). Ernst was appointed professor in 1895 but largely withdrew from active research and public-health activity. He was, in many ways, the perfect candidate to whom to hand the baton, to be the public face and chief remonstrant against antivivisectionist legislative sallies. He cared not for the task.

Ernst was rallying troops and soliciting information by correspondence, noting to William Park (1863–1939), the New York bacteriologist, that 'We are unfortunate here in being obliged to gird up our loins and fight another attempt to do away with experimentation on animals' and seeking informa-tion on the current opinions of leading antivivisectionists.[42] Replies to his letters came in, arming him with accounts of the direct benefits of diphtheria antitoxin, anaesthesia, and the like, from practising physicians. Despite Ernst's preliminary efforts, Bowditch made clear at the March hearing that there was no organized defence, but its organization would quickly be finalized. At the second hearing, Bowditch himself had been interviewed at length about the relative merits of vivisection and the extent to which medical men could be left at liberty to control and conduct their own affairs. Bowditch averred that if the laboratories of Harvard Medical School could not be entrusted to the 'control of the best men we can find' who already worked there, then it would not be possible to find anybody to meet the required degree of trust.[43] The interview meandered, Bowditch being pulled from his point, stuck in the webs created by a layman lawyer who was confused, perhaps wilfully, about the subject at hand. Asked if the author-ities at Harvard knew what went on in its laboratories, Bowditch deferred to the answer of Harvard's President, whose own testimony – that of a layman, to be sure, but a powerful one – would do the trick. The same evening, 6 March 1900, the Boston Society of Medical Sciences assembled at the St Botolph Club on Commonwealth Avenue, together comprising the Committee for the Opposition of Legislation restricting Experimentation upon Animals, (chairman Ernst), as well as the Boston Society for Medical Improvement, and the Committee on Legislation of the Massachusetts

[41] John Harley Warner, 'Ernst, Harold Clarence', in *American National Biography* (Oxford: Oxford University Press, 1999).
[42] Ernst to Park, 26 February 1900, H MS c 40, Folder 308, Box 26, WBCA.
[43] Stenographer's typescript, 'Hearing on House Bill No. 917', 6 March 1900, 13, H MS c 40 Folder 314, Box 26, WBCA.

Medical Society. Bowditch was elected Chair of the meeting and immediately announced its object: to prepare 'testimony to be used upon the proposed Bill restricting animal experimentation in Massachusetts'.[44] Of particular concern was the lumbar puncture research on children, carried out by A. H. Wentworth, which was being cast as human vivisection and which the assembled medical researchers agreed 'would be difficult to defend', 'whatever its ultimate value'.[45] Wentworth himself was present, expressing regret 'that his published account of the work was not so written as to prevent a layman from deriving an unfavorable impression', but it was clear that the assembled experts shared that unfavourable view. Their concern was that otherwise sound arguments about the value of vivisection and of their general humanitarian character would be derailed by the Bill's sponsors focusing on the spectre of human vivisection and the abuse of children in particular. While some clearly favoured Wentworth giving an account of himself, others saw no use in defending the experiments. Such outliers were a thorn in the side of the defence of a profession that did not have a coordinated code of experimental ethics; a profession that, in fact, relied on the moral fibre or character of its members to avoid unethical behaviour. Cases like Wentworth's risked upsetting the whole thing. Unsurprisingly, William Sedgwick (1855–1921), the MIT epidemiologist, mooted at this meeting the value of forming a society for the protection of biological research in Massachusetts. Bowditch concurred, also suggesting the value of 'the framing of rules governing vivisection in the Harvard Medical School'.[46] Both these ideas would ultimately come to pass, but on a much grander scale than Sedgwick and Bowditch then imagined. But the meeting to organize a remonstrance against the antivivisectionist Bill would provide a model, for the coming years, of expert community organization and mobilization.

Much of the discussion with Bowditch at the hearing earlier that afternoon had centred on the question of pain and suffering and the extent to which animals were forced to endure it for the sake of the production of knowledge, with Bowditch deflecting and justifying, but getting bogged down in the distinctions between cold-blooded and warm-blooded sensibilities, and the relative qualities of anaesthetics, curare and narcotics. In his

---

[44] Typescript of minutes, 'Boston Society of Medical Sciences', 6 March 1900, H MS c 40, Folder 321, Box 26, WBCA.

[45] For context, see Susan Lederer, 'Orphans as Guinea Pigs: American Children and Medical Experimenters, 1890–1930', in *In the Name of the Child: Health and Welfare, 1880–1940*, ed. Roger Cooter (New York: Routledge, 2013).

[46] Typescript of minutes, 'Boston Society of Medical Sciences', 6 March 1900, H MS c 40, Folder 321, Box 26, WBCA. An undated placard stating the 'Rules Regarding Animals' and signed 'Director of the Laboratory' is included in this folder, with special attention to the use of anaesthesia and animal welfare.

remonstrance at the next hearing, President Eliot brushed all this aside as irrelevant, daring to say what many physiologists could not say. Using the example of the production of diphtheria antitoxin, which took place on a grand scale at Harvard, and which caused all of the guinea pigs involved 'discomfort and pain', Eliot asked rhetorically if it was worth it. 'The question', he said, 'is whether it is worth while that animals should so serve the human race'. His positive answer was strong: 'I should go much beyond that simple affirmative, and say that I should not be able to fix a limit to the amount of suffering that animals ought to be subjected to to save one human baby. Would any of us', he asked, 'weigh the life of a thousand guinea pigs against the life of one of our children?' Moral equations that pitted humans against other animals were therefore not only invalid but in bad taste, a case of misplaced or inadequate humanity. It was here that Eliot would provide an enduring slogan for the American defenders of experimental research: 'the humanity which would prevent human suffering is a deeper and truer humanity than the humanity which would save pain or death to animals'. There was to be no compunction about it. Medical research carried out using animals was, he said, 'absolutely the most humane of human occupations, because it has prevented human suffering and death on a great scale, and because it promises to achieve in the future still greater triumphs over pain and death'. Here, distilled to its very essence, Eliot professed the humanity of medical professionals.[47]

What is more, he did so while scrupulously avoiding the question previously put to Bowditch, about the extent to which he knew what went on in Harvard's laboratories. It was not, he indicated, for him to know. How could he? Indeed, how could anyone? There was 'no authority' to permit or disallow a laboratory experiment, for the chief authority on this question was the laboratory-based expert himself. 'We may examine plumbers or dentists or physicians', Eliot said, 'because we can obtain a board competent to pass upon their qualifications; but there is no possibility of determining in that way the qualifications of the rare men who are competent to devote themselves to medical research'. Expertise was rare; its exercise was 'beneficent'.[48] Judging it by any external standard was impossible. Better, then, to acknowledge this limitation and let research take the course the researchers themselves deemed fit. As Bowditch had said, if they could not be trusted, who could?

Sedgwick also had a major impact on the Bill's fate. Gesturing at Bowditch, and referring to his glittering local, national and international

---

[47] Charles W. Eliot, 'Animal Experimentation', in *Animal Experimentation: A Series of Statements Indicating Its Value to Biological and Medical Science*, ed. Harold C. Ernst (Boston: Little, Brown, 1902), 2.
[48] Eliot, 'Animal Experimentation', 1.

reputation, he asked if it was 'necessary', or 'just', or 'right' that he should be held to be 'guilty of cruelty that he must henceforth be *licensed* like a *rumseller* or *watched* like a suspected *pickpocket* or *counterfeiter*?' To pretend to legislate against *cruelty* was to assume that cruelty was part of the modus operandi of medical experimentation, and this, with not a little class chauvinism, Sedgwick denied. The Bill, he said, was not in 'the best interests of humanity', clarifying in cross examination that far from hardening the practitioner, vivisection 'makes men more humane and tenderhearted', noting that he had himself given up shooting as 'needless slaughter'.[49] The Bill was thrown out.

When another Bill, much the same as that of 1900, came up in 1901, Ernst organized the remonstrance by himself. He had begun collecting testimony, via Sedgwick at MIT, immediately after the conclusion of the 1900 hearings, pursuing accurate information about the extent of vivisection in the State of Massachusetts and the kinds of regulations employed in the laboratories where it took place. The overwhelming majority had no rules whatsoever. At Smith College, Harris Wilder (1864–1928) stated that no rules have ever been formulated, but he assumed 'that my other teachers and myself are normally humane, and that definite laws are not necessary'.[50] At Tufts, J. S. Kingsley (1854–1929) said there were 'absolutely no rules concerning vivisection'.[51] His colleague A. Mathews enumerated the best practices there, which were in line with humane principles, but admitted that customs 'vary from time to time with the instructor until an unwritten law of precedent has been established'.[52] S. F. Clarke (1851–1928) at Williams emphasized the careful use of anaesthetics in the biological laboratory but declared 'no written rules'. Hibbert Winslow Hill (1871–1947), director of the Health Department Bacteriological Laboratory wrote that 'We have never had to formulate exact rules' and expressed gladness that there was a 'move to formulate' them.[53] At Amherst College, John M. Tyler (1875–1929) said there were 'no definite [rules] or regulations governing our laboratories'.[54] At Mount Holyoke College there were 'no specific rules, but a general understanding that vivisection is quite unnecessary in the teaching of college classes', and at Wellesley College, M. A. Wilcox formulated the rules in his reply, emphasizing 'the interests of humanity'.[55] In sum, it was evident that

---

[49] Memorandum of remarks of W. T. Sedgwick on restriction of vivisection bill, 1900, Sedgwick to Ernst, 10 April 1900, H MS c 40, Folder 309, Box 26, WBCA.
[50] Wilder to Sedgwick, 21 May 1900, H MS c 40, Folder 309, Box 26, WBCA.
[51] Kingsley to Sedgwick, 20 May 1900, H MS c 40, Folder 309, Box 26, WBCA.
[52] Mathews to Sedgwick, 22 May 1900, H MS c 40, Folder 309, Box 26, WBCA.
[53] Hill to Sedgwick, 3 May 1900, H MS c 40, Folder 309, Box 26, WBCA.
[54] Tyler to Sedgwick, 5 May 1900, H MS c 40, Folder 309, Box 26, WBCA.
[55] Wilcox to Sedgwick, 4 May 1900, H MS c 40, Folder 309, Box 26, WBCA.

researchers and instructors in biological sciences were indeed, however implicitly, asking the public to take them at their word that they were humane men. Given the ongoing pressure from antivivisectionist societies, it made no sense to continue without clear rules for everyone to follow.

Rules were quickly drawn up and posted for the Harvard Laboratories, but the opposition changed tack and, at the 1901 hearings, Bowditch was attacked for having posted them. In cross examination, Bowditch was asked why, 'considering the character of the instructors for whom the rules were made', it had seemed 'necessary to post the rules at all'. Without rules, they were asking to be taken on trust; with rules they risked advertising that trust alone was insufficient. Bowditch formulated an answer: 'Because of the new instructors who came, – it saved the constant repetition and explanation to anyone who came to the laboratory'. Nonetheless, he said, 'the spirit has *always prevailed* in the laboratory'.[56]

The result of the 1901 Bill was much the same as in 1900, being thrown out without a division. Ernst, feeling that it was pointless to do this year after year without documenting the contents of the remonstrances, compiled those for 1901 and published them in a book.[57] Here for the first time, for an American audience, were the well-rehearsed arguments of a generation. Both Bowditch and Ernst drew heavily upon English scientists, the provivisection views of T. H. Huxley in particular, and upon the arguments of Gerald Yeo's pseudonymously published *Physiological Cruelty* (1883). The great and good of Massachusetts medicine, from surgeons to physiologists, as well as clergymen, spoke of the wealth of good that came from vivisection, and the relative value of the human in the balance with other animals. Ernst closed the remonstrance with a mocking gesture: 'These presidents of great educational institutions; these representatives of the clergy, teachers of various branches of biological science, surgeons and practitioners of different beliefs; these mental, moral degenerates; these human or humane defectives – whatever epithet actually used was – rest their case in your hands'.[58] It was a scornful and resentful passage, presented in a book that captured the feeling of insult and betrayal that medical scientists and the medical community at large felt at having their best intentions second-guessed by people who knew but a little of their work. As Bowditch put it, with resignation:

That the medical profession and the higher educational institutions of the State should be called upon to defend before a legislative committee their right to study and teach does not . . . surprise any one. . . . The efforts of misguided benevolence

---

[56] Cross examination of Bowditch by French, remonstrance to Massachusetts House Bills 855 and 856, 14 March 1901, 5, H MS c 40, Folder 316, Box 26, WBCA.
[57] Ernst, *Animal Experimentation*.   [58] Ernst, *Animal Experimentation*, 176.

have ... been directed to checking the progress of medical science by interfering with one of the most important methods by which advances can be made.

It was a matter of good fortune 'for humanity' that 'these efforts have in nearly all cases been rendered futile by the sound common sense of the community'.[59]

The tone would stick, but the decision made by Ernst to publish showed a change in tactics. It put both laboratory practice and the production of knowledge on display, figuratively opening the doors that antivivisectionists often claimed to be sealed shut, and demonstrating to a lay public the passion and commitment with which these men set about vigorously defending the principles and methods of their work. It was with a degree of dismay that Ernst had to rally the community again year after year to defend these practices in the legislature. It was becoming habitual, the arguments and speeches simply being repeated, but Ernst received much flattery for his efforts. Sedgwick told him, in 1905, that Ernst reminded him of 'a good chess player moving his pieces', and David Cheever (1876–1955) congratulated him on 'the masterly manner in which you marshalled your forces, horse, foot and artillery'.[60] Horace D. Arnold (d. 1935) also used the word 'masterly', twice, in his congratulatory note.[61] It was becoming a quasi-military operation, performed with surgical precision, with Ernst as the reluctant but ever successful general. The problem was that no victory was ever final. Come the new year, there was always another Bill, always another campaign to plan. By 1906 he had clearly had his fill and refused to join the fray.

It seems to have been Sedgwick who changed his mind, impressing upon Ernst the risk of allowing the antivivisectionists' new lawyer, Samuel L. Powers (1848–1929), a free field to exploit. Sedgwick described him to Ernst as an 'extremely popular, persuasive and jolly fellow as well as an ex-congressman, a telephone lawyer and a politician of very wide influence and connections'.[62] Ernst relented, but his correspondence took on a strikingly desultory tone. To Horace Arnold he moaned, 'I am afraid that my firmness will not impress you greatly when I say that after all I am to conduct the case for the remonstrants.... As you will realize, I have reached this decision at the risk of very considerable personal inconvenience'.[63] He repeated those lines to S. H. Durgin, John McCollom, Austin Peters and W. T. Porter (1862–1949), mocking himself for failing to stick to his

---

[59] Ernst, *Animal Experimentation*, 65.
[60] Sedgwick to Ernst, 15 March 1905, H MS c 40, Folder 311, Box 26, WBCA.
[61] Cheerver to Ernst, 17 March 1905, H MS c 40, Folder 311, Box 26, WBCA.
[62] Sedgwick to Ernst, 15 February 1906, H MS c 40, Folder 312, Box 26, WBCA.
[63] Ernst to Arnold, 20 February 1906, H MS c 40, Folder 312, Box 26, WBCA.

conviction to bow out.[64] To Theobald Smith he claimed 'the right to change my mind', 'like many women', and observed that he was changing his 'to an unusual extent'. He called it the 'usual fight', the 'annual blister', the 'usual bill', and set about his task with the utmost chagrin.[65]

Most agreed to join in, but Ernst's fatigue and exasperation were shared. C. F. Hodge was ill, so wrote his remonstrance in beleaguered tone:

This discussion has been brought before the Massachusetts Legislature year after year. I have attended the hearings faithfully, thinking that surely these eagles (I am strongly tempted to call them double-back-action repeating harpies of science) would not dare bring up the matter again unless they had discovered, or thought they had discovered, some actual abuses, existing at present in some laboratory within the State. Every year they have utterly failed to show that they even thought they had discovered abuses of scientific experimentation of any sort.[66]

He also drew attention to a petition then circulating in Massachusetts, which made erroneous and de-contextualized use of a statement – by then a cliché – of Henry Bigelow (1818–90), Bowditch's predecessor at Harvard. Hodge begged to suggest 'that it is unfair to harrow up the emotions of the public today with any such antiquated, obsolete, disconnected and distorted statements'.[67] The establishment was thoroughly irritated.

The Bill was dismissed without debate, again. But the context of all these repeated excursions was changing. The opening of the Rockefeller Institute (see Chapter 5), which had a physical space by 1906, shifted the ground again back to New York. Meanwhile, Bowditch had been involved in the opening of a new front, of a nature completely different to legislative entanglements. A rumour had been abroad that the antivivisectionists were proposing to open a 'Chamber of Torture' exhibit at the St Louis World's Fair in 1904. There seemed to be no truth to it, but Bowditch was all over it, as were others, seeking assurances from the Medical Director of the Fair that no such thing should be allowed.[68] The risk of such publicity was a threat of a magnitude the establishment could not afford. If public opinion were lost, then all the parades of remonstrants in State legislatures

---

[64] Ernst to Durgin, 20 February 1906; Ernst to McCollom, 20 February 1906; Ernst to Peters, 20 February 1906; Ernst to Porter, 20 February 1906, H MS c 40, Folder 312, Box 26, WBCA.

[65] Ernst to Smith, 20 February 1906, H MS c 40, Folder 312, Box 26, WBCA.

[66] Hodge to Ernst, 25 February 1906, H MS c 40, Folder 313, Box 26, WBCA.

[67] Hodge to Ernst, 25 February 1906, H MS c 40, Folder 313, Box 26, WBCA.

[68] Bowditch to F. J. Lutz, 4 February 1904; 8 February 1904; Baumgarten to Bowditch, 12 February 1904; Keen to Bowditch, 15 February 1904; Tuhoske to Bowditch, 15 February 1904; Hodge to Ernst, 25 February 1906, H MS c 40, Folder 307, Box 26, WBCA.

would count for little. It was a period when the medical community were acutely aware of the need for continued vigilance and the maintenance of energy about the defence of their profession, yet they were showing clear signs of being worn down. After the 1906 hearings in Boston, that lively lawyer about whom Sedgwick had warned, wrote personally to Ernst, suggesting it was time for a compromise. 'At the close of our hearing', he wrote, 'Bowditch came to me and suggested that he thought the time had come when the friends of the proposed legislation and those opposing it ought to get together and agree upon some bill which would be reasonable and mutually satisfactory'. He called for co-operation with 'men representing the medical profession'. He proposed forming a committee to meet in the summer a draw up a bill that would meet with both sides' approval. The moment of compromise – that moment that Michael Foster had long since warned against – was upon them. Ernst put the matter to his Committee for the Opposition of Legislation, who rebuffed it.[69] It seems implausible, given the preceding years, that Bowditch had intimated such a compromise, but the ad hoc affairs of the medical community in defence of vivisection were making no headway. At this moment, a new figure emerged, injecting fresh vigour and, importantly, a bigger vision. Walter B. Cannon, who would be Bowditch's successor at Harvard, declared himself 'ready to add my shot in the bombardment'.[70]

---

[69] Powers to Ernst, 12 April 1906; Ernst to Powers, 7 May 1906, H MS c 40, Folder 313, Box 26, WBCA.

[70] Cannon to Ernst, 22 February 1906, H MS c 40, Folder 313, Box 26, WBCA.

4   Paget's Public

Renewed Public Engagement

Back in England, if the Association for the Advancement of Medicine by Research had largely fallen silent in the 1890s, then it re-emerged as an important voice in the battle for public opinion on the matter of vivisection somewhat earlier than has been previously thought. Attention has tended towards the 'Brown Dog Affair' and the Second Royal Commission (about which more below) in precipitating a more visible presence for the AAMR, but the Committee had actually elected to emerge from anonymous activity as early as 1900. The Secretary of the Association, Stephen Paget, had perceived a need to put the arguments in favour of experimental research to the public, and specifically used his experience with the AAMR to make his case in a book length study to be 'written for general reading'. The book, styled simply *Experiments on Animals*, was introduced by Lister, who took the opportunity to decry the 'ignorance' of 'well-meaning persons' who denied the 'greatness of the benefits' that experimental research had 'conferred upon mankind'.[1] The book's defence revealed how the Act was administered and also answered specific charges of the various antivivisection societies. Paget was setting himself up as the expert who knew both sides equally. He did no scientific research of his own, but he researched antivivisectionist literature with some thoroughness, calling for a Royal Commission into *this*, as well as into experimentation itself. He was seeing the road ahead, understanding that fertile ground for a defence of research lay in denunciation of the opponents of science. A general tenor of ridicule, put forward by men and women of the *right sort*, could be the ideal vehicle for a presentation of what he perceived to be the true terms of humanity or mercy. As Paget himself put it in the third edition of his book, 'where, in all

---

[1] The book went through many editions and was also published separately in the United States. Stephen Paget, *Experiments on Animals* (London: T. Fisher Unwin, 1900/ New York: William Wood, 1900), xi–xii. The two first editions are identical.

this confusion', in this parade of 'discordant societies', in this 'Falstaff's army of the osteopath, and the fruitarian, and the *anti* this, that and the other', can 'we find the ethical argument? Mercy is admirable, but I will wait till mercy and truth are met together'.[2] Such would be the leitmotiv of the early twentieth-century defence of research.

If Paget's book betrayed a cockiness derived from the success of AAMR activities behind the scenes, the relative quietness of antivivisectionism would be shattered by a new voice in 1903. Emilia Augusta Louise Lind af Hageby (1878–1963) – Lizzie – signed up for classes at University College London in 1902 and soon thereafter denounced the practices of some of physiology's leading lights as borne on a wave of heartless cruelty and horrific mirth. Her enduring fame stems from the libel trial (which she lost) occasioned by her co-authorship of *Shambles of Science* in 1903, which touched off the 'Brown Dog Affair': the claim that Professors Bayliss (1860–1924) and Starling (1866–1927) had experimented upon a dog in a scene of unanaesthetized and torturous 'fun'. I do not want to dwell on the Brown Dog Affair, in the main because it has already received significant historiographical treatment from others.[3] That treatment has, by and large, focused on the event's significance for the antivivisection movement and for animal representation, of which Lind af Hageby would come to play a leading part. My interest in it concerns the scientific reaction to the trial, the renewed focus on animal experimentation at the level of government, and the subsequent organization of the defence of medical research using animals at an institutional level involving both scientific and lay figures. The Brown Dog Affair's importance, for the purposes of this story, lies in what came after it. After all, one could sum up the Affair from the point of view of the medical scientists as a rather simple victory against a published falsehood. Bayliss won his libel suit, *Shambles of Science* was withdrawn and pulped, reputations were upheld, and those of antivivisectionists were tarnished. There was a public outcry, detailed in Lansbury's classic account, which was a large causal factor in the appointment of a second Royal Commission to enquire into the subject of vivisection. The feeling among the scientific community was that a much greater defensive attitude needed to be adopted. The threat of future such public disturbances and associated

[2] Stephen Paget, *Experiments on Animals*, 3rd edn (New York: William Wood, 1907), 330–31.
[3] Coral Lansbury, *The Old Brown Dog: Women, Workers, and Vivisection in Edwardian England* (Madison: University of Wisconsin Press, 1985); Ben Garlick, 'Not All Dogs Go to Heaven, Some Go to Battersea: Sharing Suffering and the "Brown Dog Affair"', *Social & Cultural Geography*, 16 (2015): 798–820; Hilda Kean, 'An Exploration of the Sculptures of Greyfriars Bobby, Edinburgh, Scotland, and the Brown Dog, Battersea, South London, England', *Society & Animals*, 11 (2003): 353–73.

media events seemed plausible given that there was nothing to stop the circumstances of it coming about again.

Starling's Flock

The second Royal Commission on the question of vivisection was appointed in 1906. It would have a troubled course. Taking evidence for two years, the Commission was de-railed by the deaths of commissioners that delayed the final report for four years. By the time that report came out in 1912, by and large reconfirming the medical establishment in its experimental purpose and extolling the virtues of the licensing system that had been established in 1876, things had already moved on apace. There had been, from the moment of the Commission's appointment, an escalation of strategic organization within the experimental community to make sure that medical research was at no point wrong footed by antivivisectionist organization.

The Physiological Society, which, as we have seen, had come into existence as a sort of drawing room committee of eminent associates of Darwin, with a front line of professional young-gun specialists, spawned a new committee of its own explicitly to deal with the Royal Commission. It was to co-ordinate the whole landscape of professional organizations within the medical establishment in order to feed witnesses and testimony to the Commission and in order to streamline channels of communication. It was a striking assertion – even an arrogation – of organizational authority. At a stroke, the Physiological Society created a new committee that would rally the Royal Society, the Royal College of Physicians, the Royal College of Surgeons, the British Medical Association, the Association for the Advancement of Medicine by Research, the Pathological Society, the Neurological Society, the Royal Veterinary College 'and other bodies'. This would become known as Professor Starling's Committee.[4] Those societies sent delegates to Starling's Committee, which appointed an executive committee to manage the 'different aspects' of the subject, carefully selecting specific personnel to be supplied as expert witnesses before the Commission. Starling was completely up front about all of this in his own testimony, given over three days at the end of 1906. Yet he insisted that the 'sole aim of the committee is not to present any given cause, but to send up before the Commission those men who are specially acquainted with different aspects of the question'. This seems disingenuous, given that the medical establishment's 'cause' was well defined.[5]

---

[4] Physiological Society minutes, 12 May 1906, Physiological Society, Committee Minutes 1889–1912, SA/PHY/B.1/3, Wellcome Library, London.
[5] UK Parliament, Appendix to the First Report of the Commissioners, C. 3326 (1907), 129.

Starling was questioned specifically on this by Sir William Church (1837–1928) (who would become the President of the Royal Society of Medicine in 1908, while the Commission was still sitting), so it might be thought that the exchange was one between allies. Church asked Starling if his testimony had met with the approval of the societies his Committee coordinated and he answered in the affirmative, if with qualification: 'In so far as the societies have delegated their power to the delegates on the committee'. But he was sure that his testimony would find 'general agreement' among the whole medical community that his offshoot of the Physiological Society was managing. Practically, this meant two things. (1) Professor Starling himself represented the aggregate opinion of medical research *in toto* and was its semi-official spokesman. His testimony – about which, more below – therefore carried the seal of approval and weight of authority of a powerful collective lobby. (2) Testimony before the Royal Commission was effectively managed and controlled by Starling's Committee, which meant, given the Committee's connections across the landscape of medical societies, that the message would be consistent, surprise-free and wholly unmoved by any line of questioning that was sympathetic to the antivivisection cause. The mistakes of 1876, such as Klein's reckless testimony about anaesthetics, would not be made again.

By no means were all of the Commissioners automatically on the side of medical research by experimentation, and perhaps the most important exchange in Starling's testimony was that with Sir William Collins (1859–1946). Collins had himself been a surgeon, but he was known for his anti-vaccination opinions (a liberal, he opposed compulsion, but he also cast doubt on Jennerian methods), which had led him away from medicine and towards politics. In general, anti-vaccinationism and antivivisectionism tended to align, so Starling may have felt wary of Collins' examination. Collins was, in fact, not an antivivisectionist, but he was in favour of more stringent restrictions concerning what happened to animals under anaesthesia and of limiting the remit of medical researchers to define exceptions to the rule of experimenting with anaesthetic.[6] From Starling's point of view, therefore, Collins wished to shackle science. The exchange went to the core of the medical establishment's argument that vivisection was a practice of humanitarianism and a marker, par excellence, of civilization.

Starling had asserted that 'It is the greatest asset which a nation can have, to have among itself a number of men endowed with ... "mere curiosity"'. He had explicitly argued, as a good Darwinian (and calling on

---

[6] Arthur Salusbury MacNalty, *Sir William Collins, Surgeon and Statesman* (London: Chadwick Trust, 1949), 24–7.

Darwin's endorsement of experimental research in physiology before the Royal Commission of 1876), that physiology in particular could not be utilitarian in a pure sense and could not be fenced in by those who wished to limit experimentation to research that had direct utilitarian applications. Physiology was only utilitarian in the sense that all science was utilitarian, representing 'a phase in man's activities in the struggle for existence'. The acquisition of knowledge tended towards a decrease in suffering but research could not be predicated on this outcome. Science led by 'pure curiosity' led to an 'addition to our knowledge as a whole, and its effects may be to change the whole of the applications of that knowledge to man's needs'. This was in line with Darwin's revised edition of *Descent*, and a recapitulation of the experiment-as-practice-of-sympathy argument that had been honed by the previous generation. It was precisely this that Collins wished to interrogate. Was not 'some qualification . . . required to that as regards moral or sentimental considerations?' Starling was not sure what the question meant. Pressing again, Collins asked if it were 'not a fact that, among the grounds for not using man for the purpose of vivisection, are moral grounds?' and again Starling seemed confused. He answered: 'Yes, I suppose they are. I do not quite know what your definition of moral grounds is.'

Collins was trying to get Starling to admit that putting everything else second to the pursuit of knowledge would risk humans being used for involuntary experiments precisely upon these grounds. He was probing just how far the idea of curiosity as an asset to the nation could be pushed before it became a vice and a risk to the very fabric of civilization. 'Would that which would otherwise be a crime', Collins asked, 'be justifiable on the ground of the pursuit of knowledge?'. Starling's reply might have been lifted directly from the *Descent*, such was its orthodox Darwinism. 'I have tried to make out', he said, 'that the pursuit of knowledge is entirely for the advance of the race, and the evolution of the race is associated with the development of the highest social feelings; and such employment of your fellow creatures would be anti-social'. For Starling, the pursuit of knowledge was a 'feature of this evolution of social feeling'. Collins did not understand, seeing the question of morals and the pursuit of knowledge as separate things. Starling clarified again: 'What you call the moral feeling and the pursuit of knowledge are both parts of the evolution of the social feeling of the community'.[7]

[7] UK Parliament, Appendix to the First Report of the Commissioners, C. 3326 (1907), 128–9, 131.

Thus the Darwinian argument about the evolution of sympathy and of scientific practice as exemplary of this evolutionary adaptation was carried into the twentieth century, not as argument, but as well-rehearsed fact. In order to understand the strategic operation that followed, it is essential to understand just how entrenched Starling's position had become. Whereas the previous generation had spent their time making and reinforcing this argument, embodying it and practising it, literally feeling their way towards a new embodied experience of humanity, this generation of British medical researchers took it as a given and presented it as such. A great deal of energy had been exerted in connecting Darwin's intellectual contribution to a practical application of it. A rhetorical argument against it could not contradict the lived experience of medical research. Starling, an exemplary representative of this community, was confused by Collins' questioning because it was alien to his affective practices – his emotional, intellectual and practical way of doing his job and his appreciation of the value of that job in the world. The science of sympathy was, to its practitioners, *real*. What was needed, therefore, was acknowledgement of this reality, of scientists as an evolutionary saltation, and of medical research as an expression of advanced and highly civilized social feelings. Starling had to concede that he could find no fault with 'the lay mind' that 'looks with some anxiety on all experiments on living animals', but only because the lay mind was 'convinced that cruelty is practised'. The people who spread this message were the problem, for the people 'who believe these statements' were 'quite justified in feeling strongly about it'.[8] The problem, for Starling and his flock was that such statements were untrue. Thus, the British medical-scientific community looked for endorsements beyond their own community, to establish their reality as *the* reality. In Edwardian Britain, traction on matters such as this was still gained by seeking out the support of aristocrats, political leaders, the church and society ladies. If these people could be persuaded to say, publicly, that yes, the humanity of medical science was the *true* expression of humanity, then this reality would stand a better chance of becoming real for all. Social and political difficulties, in the fantasy of a successful lay campaign, would melt away.

Stephen Paget and Research Defence Society Strategy

The medical-scientific establishment's approach to the Royal Commission was brilliantly contrived to ensure success before Parliament. But insofar as they set out to persuade Parliament to let sleeping dogs lie and be cut,

[8] UK Parliament, Appendix to the First Report of the Commissioners, C. 3326 (1907), 131.

a clear need to win over public support to the cause had re-emerged. Even if the medical community could easily sway a public enquiry, it nevertheless took a great deal of energy, time and money. Starling and his peers across the research community would have much preferred to be left alone to get on with their jobs. Thus, a whole new communication strategy had to be carved out, so that scientists might get their message across to polite society, and from there to the population at large. The coordination of this strategy was also better handled by parties beyond the world of scientific practice, lest this too drain the energy of medical research and divert its attention to the detriment of the pursuit of knowledge. Hence the need for the Research Defence Society (RDS).

What was the RDS? I focus here on the emergence and early career of this society, with special focus on its strategic planning of the defence of medical research for which it was founded. But the RDS had a long and important life. It existed until 2008 – a century of work – before merging with the Coalition for Medical Progress and adopting a new name: Understanding Animal Research.[9] Its roots, in turn, were in the Association for the Advancement of Medical Research and the Physiological Society (see Chapter 2), appearing after a generation of experience of defending medicine against antivivisection activity replete with fully formed strategies for defence. It also had connections to Ernest Starling's Committee for collecting evidence to present to the second Royal Commission on Vivisection, which was active principally between 1906 and 1908 (finally concluding in 1912). The men attached to these various organizations tended to pass fluidly from one to the other, but one man in particular was central to the continuity of strategic thinking in the defence of research, allowing the RDS to begin with a firm course of action in mind. This was the surgeon Stephen Paget, son of the even more famous surgeon and pathologist James (Figure 4.1).

Stephen Paget founded the RDS in 1908. With his illustrious father James, he had been on the front line of the defence of experimental medicine against antivivisection for many years, as secretary of the Association for the Advancement of Medicine by Research, but his new pressure group employed novel tactics.[10] Relying on the financial contributions of the lay public, Paget sought to protect medical science, and particularly the spirit of innovation through animal experimentation, by manipulating public opinion through association with non-medical society figures. Unlike in the

---

[9] Bates dedicates chapter 6 of *Anti-Vivisection and the Profession of Medicine* to a simple history of the RDS's work, with the years from foundation to the First World War taking up pages 135–41.

[10] Stephen Paget was appointed secretary of the AAMR in May 1886, while his father was still chairman. See AAMR Minutes, 41.

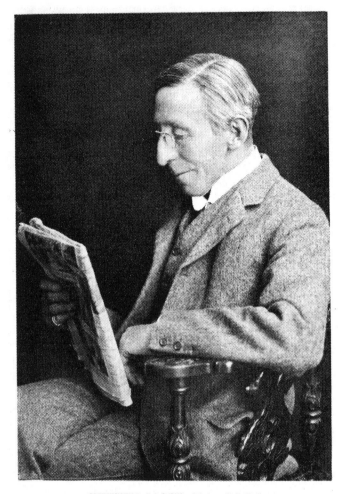

STEPHEN PAGET, M.A., F.R.C.S.
(Founder of the Research Defence Society).

Figure 4.1 Stephen Paget, founder of the Research Defence Society. Wellcome Library, London. Attribution 4.0 International (CC BY 4.0).

USA, where the formal cause of medical science would come to be strictly limited to those with medical expertise, Paget understood that the British case required champions among the chattering classes. As he told Walter Cannon at Harvard, in the English fight against antivivisection, 'a doctor counts one, a layman counts two, a lady counts three, and a cleric counts four'.[11] While much of the RDS campaign literature relied upon medical expertise, it was in the translation of medical language for a popular audience that the society sought success. In focus here is the practical application of Paget's rationale about the relative importance of lay influence.

The dynamics of engagement here were layered: medical-scientific interests were received and interpreted by the RDS, mobilized and distributed to attract lay support, and in turn used to combat a particularly strident vein of lay opposition, especially among women, to experimental medicine and to vivisection in particular. Thus, the public battle for 'medical progress' took place almost entirely among non-medical circles. A central motif of this was the orchestration and direction of emotions about medical research, along clear gender lines. Antivivisectionism was characterized as feminine hysteria or overblown sentimentalism, aimed at the preservation (oddly enough, for a movement otherwise considered progressive) of old models of religious morality and compassion. The society women of the RDS, on the other hand, were portrayed as more sensibly in thrall to the rationalism of science and its predominantly masculine innovative endeavours to end human suffering.

The RDS came to life on 27 January 1908, at a meeting of Professor Starling's Committee at Harley Street, London. The meeting marked both an informal handover of power from Starling and a formal endeavour to institutionalize the defence of research. It came with a golden hello of £100 from the Physiological Society and £85 from Starling's committee, and with explicit instructions to Paget – appointed as Honorary Secretary as the first order of business – to secure premises, headed stationery and a press-cuttings service; to circulate letters of invitation to people who 'might help', and to assist those who would stand on behalf of medicine wherever animal experimentation was to be debated in public. It was resolved that Paget should be immediately dispatched to Parliament to lobby MPs. And the newly formed RDS promptly set about finding an eminent layman to serve as President.[12] Lord Cromer (1841–1917), the former Consul-General of Egypt and ardent anti-suffragist, agreed to serve in this capacity, and was instructed to announce the foundation of the society in a letter to major newspapers. He would later write that he

[11] This appraisal was quoted by Cannon in a letter to Lee, based on correspondence between Paget and Cannon. Cannon to Lee, 8 December 1908, H MS c 40, Folder 339, Box 28, WBCA.

[12] RDS Minute of 27 January 1908, Committee minutes from inauguration of RDS, SA/RDS/C/1: Box 2, Wellcome Library London. Assessing the historical value of money is notoriously difficult, but based on the MeasuringWorth.com calculation of 'project' value – that is, total assets or net worth of, say, a company – £185 might amount to as much £195 100 in 2018 terms.

accepted the role because he 'felt strongly that the Vivisectionists, and not their opponents, were the true humanitarians'. Only they were visionary enough to understand a calculus of suffering at the level of society. The success of science 'would connote the decrease of premature mortality and the mitigation of suffering'. He understood that scientists' efforts to 'enlighten the public ... might perhaps in some degree be aided by association with those who, like myself, realised the vast importance of the issue at stake, albeit they could bring no special scientific acquirements to bear on the various technical points'.[13] Cromer had it in a nutshell. When his notice announcing the foundation was published, on 25 April 1908, the society already boasted 800 members. A month later that number had risen to 1200, including 100 ladies.[14] By December, Paget was boasting of 1700 members, including 170 ladies, and by the anniversary of the RDS's inauguration there were 2200 members, including 250 ladies.[15] Given the minimum yearly subscription of five shillings, one can easily grasp the immediate and resounding success of the RDS in terms of securing financial backing – some £550 in subscriptions alone, exclusive of large individual donations.

The RDS Committee clearly saw the successful scientific management of the Royal Commission to be a potentially useful strategic aid in its campaign, and its early efforts at publishing involved the repackaging of various pieces of testimony from the Royal Commission with the aim of engaging a 'popular scientific audience' for the driest of parliamentary publications.[16] These included the evidence of Lord Justice Fletcher Moulton (1844–1921), Colonel David Bruce (1855–1931) on Malta fever, and Professor Cushny (1866–1926) on pharmacology.[17] Fletcher Moulton is worth our attention precisely because of the role he carved out for himself as an eminent layperson, a man of learning, a politician, a Lord Justice, but certainly not a man of medical training himself. He told the Royal Commission that he had 'realised for many years' that the question of

[13] Lord Cromer, 'Introduction', in *For and Against Experiments on Animals: Evidence before the Royal Commission on Vivisection*, ed. Stephen Paget (London: H. K. Lewis, 1912), xii.

[14] Copy of letter published in newspapers, re establishment of RDS, 24 April 1908, RDS Occasional Publications and Printed Papers, SA/RDS/G/1/1:Box 13, Wellcome Library, London.

[15] RDS, Birmingham Branch minute book, SA/RDS/C/15: Box 6, 6, 13.

[16] RDS Minute of 3 March 1908, Committee minutes from inauguration of RDS, SA/RDS/C/1: Box 2, Wellcome Library London. This ultimately culminated in a weighty volume of digested testimony and other essays: Paget, *For and Against Experiments*. Despite its title, scant attention was given to those 'against'.

[17] Research Defence Society, *Evidence of Lord Justice Fletcher Moulton before the Royal Commission on Vivisection* (London: Macmillan, 1908); Colonel David Bruce, *The Extinction of Malta Fever (A Lesson in the Use of Animal Experimentation)* (London: Macmillan, 1908); A. R. Cushny, 'Vivisecton and Medicine: Have Experiments on Animals Advanced Therapeutics' (1908). RDS Occasional Publications and Printed Papers, SA/RDS/G/1/4, 6, 11:Box 13, Wellcome Library, London.

vivisection would come to be scrutinized by Parliament, precisely because the work of scientists had become 'more and more beyond the ken of the ordinary public', which nevertheless continued to exercise a perceived 'right and ... duty of controlling everything that goes on in the kingdom'. He styled himself an 'interpreter', a man to 'explain and justify' medical research. No wonder the RDS would come to make use of him. And later, of course, Fletcher Moulton would become the first chair of the Medical Research Committee, about which more below. He represented the 'curative sciences' and the research that supported them as being constantly confronted with pain, with the sole desire of diminishing it in the present and, importantly, *in the future*. This aspect of the debate was, he reflected, often ignored by the opponents of vivisection. And, he thought, it took a truly humane heart to be a man who would inflict present pain to save a greater preponderance of future pain, as opposed to the short-sighted 'tender-hearted' type, who would prevent the present pain and, by so doing, directly cause 'preventable pain on ... an enormous scale' in the future. The opponents of vivisection, he mused, were only capable of contemplating pain in a narrow sense, and their opposition was based on 'the effect of their emotions of the contemplation of pain'. They opposed the pain caused in experiments by, say, Lister, because they could not conceive of the 'prevented pain' or make it 'present to their minds'. Only the 'inflicted pain' struck 'their imagination' and thus they denounced the likes of Lister with 'the best of motives'. Yet they were ultimately wrong, making humanitarian pronouncements while labouring under a defect of too much emotion. The true humanitarian could 'regard the more distant consequences', free of any immediate emotional reaction to the infliction of pain in the laboratory.[18] It is hard to imagine a more succinct digest of the Darwinian/Spencerian view of the scientist as emotionally superior, his humane professions carrying the weight of a higher evolutionary stage of human social evolution.[19]

This would be the leitmotiv of RDS rhetoric, but there was more to Paget's motivations. Although there is a good record of evidence of the RDS's early activities in its minute books and printed pamphlets, the most revealing source of information are Paget's letters to medical scientists in the USA. In these epistles we find Paget candid, enthusiastic, rather pompous, sometimes self-congratulatory, often cloyingly sycophantic. Although the Americans used Paget as a guide as to how *not* to act,

---

[18] UK Parliament, Appendix to the Third Report of the Commissioners, C. 3757 (1907), 251–3.

[19] See, in particular, the Spencerian view on the detachment of highly evolved minds from immediate aesthetic sympathetic reactions. 'Species of Compassion: Aesthetics, Anaesthetics and Pain in the Physiological Laboratory', *19: Interdisciplinary Studies in the Long Nineteenth Century*, 15 (2012).

especially in terms of the relationship between medical expertise and lay support, Paget presented himself as a source of inspiration to the American campaign. A minute of 31 March 1908 noted that Paget had already written to Drs Millican (Chicago) and Cushing (1869–1939) (Baltimore), 'urging the formation in America of a Society similar to the Research Defence Society and in close touch with it'.[20] The RDS came into existence before the Council for the Defense of Medical Research in the USA (see the following chapter), and was an impetus for the American medical establishment to formally organize a defence initiative, but the similarity largely ended there. Though medical research met with the same type of antivivisection campaign on both sides of the Atlantic – indeed, they often met with exactly the same opponents, since both Lind af Hageby and Stephen Coleridge (1854–1936) went on American antivivisection lecture tours – they adopted entirely different strategies to combat it in these years. In England, this built upon the experience of the preceding generation of gentlemanly science and the realities of a medical research practice that was already subject to government oversight in the form of licences for experimentation. In the USA, it was built upon a fractured experience of legislative challenges at the State level, and of medical research as an essentially private (and privately funded) professional activity. Emerging at almost exactly the same time, the RDS was essentially a medically steered lay organization to mobilize favourable lay public opinion and outshout the lay opinion of antivivisectionists. The American organization would be entirely professional, with a mind to direct education of the public, quiet manipulation of the press, and a forceful professionalized legal opposition to any form of legislative inroads against experimentation.

By the summer of 1908, Paget was enthusiastically writing to George H. Simmons (1852–1937), the editor of the *Journal of the American Medical Association*, about the triumphant launch of the RDS and of its character. By that point, Paget was boasting of 1400 members, including 140 ladies. The RDS, he reported, was establishing branches, all of which were on board with the scattergun strategy of defence: 'we are getting out more leaflets as fast as we can; and we are watching the newspapers, magazines, etc., and writing letters and articles in them. Also, we have a debater, who will go to any debate and speak; and we must get more men like him'. It was clear, even at this very early stage, that the most important factor for Paget in the battle for public sentiment was the character and reputation of the RDS membership. 'We have had a wonderful welcome', he told Simmons. 'Leaders of science, Bishops, Deans and Canons, Lords and Ladies, city

---

[20] RDS Minute of 31 March 1908, Committee minutes from inauguration of RDS, SA/RDS/C/1: Box 2, Wellcome Library London.

men, poor country doctors, engineers, teachers – they have all come! Study the list of our vice-presidents. Was there ever a more goodly list?'[21] Paget made it sound haphazard – a success despite a lack of organizational prowess – declaring, 'We have no rules! we haven't had time to make any!' The reason for the success, in his opinion, was simple:

The plain fact is that public opinion is beginning to be *sick* of Anti-vivisection societies. There are sixteen or more of these societies.... They squabble, and rant, and bully, and pervert facts, and use virulent language – and people are just tired of them, and thankful to have *our* Society. It is not so much love of science that has brought in our members, but love of fair play and common honesty, and approval of a society sticking up for an unpopular cause.[22]

Could there have been a more stereotypical evaluation of the way in which English public opinion functioned? Paget painted the RDS as an under-dog, manfully proceeding in the spirit of sporting decency, and winning friends and influence accordingly. The RDS message, which was never much more than a rehearsal of prevailing rhetoric about the overwhelm-ing benefits of vivisection for humanity, was amplified by the status of those now delivering that message. The support of aristocrats, the clergy and notable ladies, was a social guarantee of honesty and civilization. It was, moreover, a guarantee of emotional maturity in dealing with a difficult subject. It was on these terms, on the difference between elite lay emotional maturity and the sentimental vulnerability of the masses, that the battle took place.

Paget's own view on precisely who were the targets of RDS messaging and campaigning was inconsistent, even incoherent. He repeatedly informed his American colleagues that the better educated members of society were thoroughly behind the RDS cause, and he contemptibly maligned antivivisectionists, who, having given up trying to win over public opinion among the educated, turned their attention to courting 'the masses'.[23] Yet Paget also targeted this group, with all the paternalistic contempt for the uneducated that he could muster. He told Cannon that 'Our problem over here is not with the educated folk, but with the uneducated, what some people call the Masses. We want to "get at the

---

[21] Paget's letter to Simmons was forwarded to Cannon at Harvard. Simmons to Cannon, 20 August 1908. Simmons was deeply persuaded and tried to push Cannon at Harvard to follow suit and get laymen onto the CDMR. As the next chapter details, this simply made no sense to Cannon and his influential colleagues. Simmons to Cannon, 26 August 1908, H MS c 40, Box 28, Folder 333: 1908–9 correspondence with George H. Simmons re Council on the Defense of Medical Research, WBCA.

[22] Simmons to Cannon, 20 August 1908, Box 28, Folder 333: 1908–9 corres with George H. Simmons re Council on the Defense of Medical Research, WBCA.

[23] Paget to Henry James Jr, 13 February 1914, Folder 7, Box 6, FA142, Anti-vivisection Activities, RUR, RAC.

masses", and this is easier said than done'.[24] While Paget thought that the majority of the press were 'solid on our side', he knew that the 'yellow papers' were not. *The Star*, *The Morning Leader* and *The Daily News* could not be counted on, but their importance was dismissed because of their price (half a penny), which marked them out for the gutter.[25] Yet the method for reaching the masses was to compete in precisely this realm, through 'really popular leaflets or handbills, regular little tracts' that engaged in the kind of insubstantial sloganizing that characterized antivivisection.[26]

Quite why Paget felt the need to reach this group at all is mysterious. It was clear that he did not feel there was a genuine debate to be had with antivivisectionists, and he was borderline complacent about the support of a public opinion that might be said to 'count'. He understood antivivisectionism not be an earnest cause, but a case of institutional inertia overseen by the unscrupulous. There were, he told Henry James Jr (1879–1947)[27], the business manager of the Rockefeller Institute in New York, 'heaps of money' in the antivivisection societies, and those societies were therefore obliged to spend it. Hence the regulatory law, the slew of government reports and commissions of enquiry, 'have never established any sort or kind of peace or equilibrium'. While the 'Brown Dog case, and the result of Miss Lind af Hageby's action, and the defeat of Sir Frederick Banbury's Dog Protection Bill, and the flight of the Secretary of Coleridge's Society, taking £5000 with him; and, above all, the steady and successful work of the Research Defence Society' had all contributed to a certain desperation among antivivisectionist activists, Paget nevertheless saw 'no end to the fight' so long as there was 'money to be spent'. In the end, Paget's motivation seemed to be rooted in a sense of moral opprobrium about the insidious influence of untruths, not only on the reputations of medical scientists, but on the outlook of the 'masses' per se. As he told James Jr,

I think the real difficulty may be put very plainly. We have had, for more than thirty years, a small number of people who are liars. These lies and half lies have been eagerly swallowed by a host of people who do not understand how false they are. These falsehoods have been passionately asserted by paid lecturers, incessantly, all over the country, and have been distributed in tons of leaflets. They have taken of late years a very gross form.... I do not know any other word but lying for deliberate attempts to make ignorant people believe what the speaker or writer knows to be false.[28]

---

[24] Paget to Cannon, 23 January 1910, H MS c 40, Box 29, Folder 350, WBCA.
[25] Paget to Cannon, n.d. [1910], H MS c 40, Box 29, Folder 350, WBCA.
[26] Paget to Cannon, 23 January 1910, H MS c 40, Box 29, Folder 350, WBCA.
[27] Henry James III, son of William James (1842–1910), the pioneer psychologist.
[28] Paget to Henry James Jr, 13 February 1914, Folder 7, Box 6, FA142, Anti-vivisection Activities, RUR, RAC.

Implicitly, therefore, the RDS not only protected experimental medicine from attack, but it also acted as a paternalistic guardian of the gullible masses. Were they of particular value to the cause? It hardly seems so. This element, coupled with the fact that the RDS was explicitly a lay society, turned the campaign into something like moral suasion or, fancifully, social control. In 1913, for example, Paget sent a note to Simon Flexner, director of the Rockefeller, regarding his work combating meningitis, along with a selection of RDS pamphlets. He remarked: 'We are pegging away quietly, over here, at the humble business of fighting anti-vivisection! It is strange, that such work as yours should need defence!'[29] One can detect Paget's fatigue with such a mission, as he sighed to James Jr that his society was 'pegging away, educating people, and nailing lies to the counter'. Although 'educated folk' were tired of antivivisection, 'there is a lot of educating still to be done amongst non-educated folk'.[30]

Eminent Ladies

Time and again, the RDS saw material advantage in drawing attention to the support it received (having actively pursued it) from eminent society women. The involvement of women at an organizational level was pronounced, particularly in some of the RDS branch societies, which the RDS had aimed to establish from the outset.[31] The Kensington branch, for example was founded in May 1910 by a meeting of seventeen well-to-do society figures, nine of whom were women. This number included Alice Corthorn, MB, who had become an experimental expert on plague while stationed in India. Paget made special mention of her 'splendid' work in his *Experiments on Animals*. But Corthorn was something of an exception as a female medical professional among the RDS ranks. The rest of the assemblage were more characteristic. The meeting took place in the drawing room of 'Mrs Arthur Somervell' – Edith – the wife of the celebrated composer. Many of the other ladies are difficult to identify, but one, Marion Black-Hawkins, unmarried, wrote about the keeping of unusual pets, such as snakes and spiders, and once claimed to have befriended a wasp.[32]

---

[29] Paget to Flexner, re meningitis, 19 May 1913, Flexner Paget correspondence, Reel 86, FA746, Series 1 Simon Flexner Paper; Subseries 1.2 Rockefeller Institute for Medical Research, Simon Flexner Papers (American Philosophical Society), RAC

[30] Paget to Henry James Jr, 13 February 1914, Folder 7, Box 6, FA142, Anti-vivisection Activities, RUR, RAC.

[31] RDS Minute of 14 April 1908, Committee minutes from inauguration of RDS, SA/RDS/C/1: Box 2, Wellcome Library London.

[32] *Luton Times and Advertiser*, 9 July 1909; *Nottingham Evening Post*, 8 December 1913; *Aberdeen Journal*, 4 May 1914. These references were located thanks to 'St Mary Bourne

Animal interests tended to align either in favour or against vivisection, but in the main the more well-to-do tended to fall in behind the cause of medical research.

The female voice was deployed as an authoritative affective weight to determine the balance of arguments between antivivisectionists and scientists. The strategy was quite deliberate. Antivivisection was characterized by its mistrust of scientific evidence and of scientific rhetoric. Denial of cruelty, explanation of the technicalities of anaesthesia, descriptions of humanitarian applications of research, and so on, when they came from practising scientists themselves, made no difference at all to antivivisectionist cant. Even in direct correspondence in the pages of the national newspapers, having the better of the argument counted for nothing if the rhetoric of, say, Stephen Coleridge of the National Anti-Vivisection Society is anything to go by. Whereas American medical scientists had the conviction of being right and the confidence that their authority would count for something in the court of public opinion, the RDS had an explicit understanding that one could not reap the fruit of trust from the seeds of mistrust. They therefore appealed to and employed lay voices, especially eminent female lay voices, where trustworthiness was not so easily gainsaid in public.

In late 1908 and early 1909, for example, an argument ran in *The Times* between Stephen Coleridge, Victor Horsley (1857–1916) and Dudley Buxton (1855–1931) about the technicalities of anaesthetic dosage in George Washington Crile's (1864–1943) experiments on surgical shock. The two scientists, Horsley and Buxton, were at pains to show how Coleridge had wilfully misinterpreted and misreported testimony given before the Royal Commissioners. Important here is that Coleridge had made his accusations of cruelty in a circular letter sent to the Vice-Presidents of the RDS. The RDS mobilized its response in the press, compiled the correspondence into its own circular, and superadded a copy of a letter sent by reply to Coleridge from the Duchess of Montrose. Montrose – Violet Graham – was a prominent philanthropist, concerned, as was Coleridge, with the welfare of children. But she was also a leading anti-suffragist whose views were based upon a concern about the welfare of the state if voting powers were to be bestowed upon such a wealth of impressionable inexperience. It was not a simple recapitulation of the paternalist view of the franchise, so much as a class-based appreciation of the myriad ways that women had been held in check by barriers to education, professions and society per se. In Montrose's view,

Goes to War', https://stmarybournegoestowar.net/tag/black-hawkins-family/, accessed 7 May 2019.

Coleridge's antivivisectionism, and implicitly also Cobbe's and Lind af Hageby's, played and preyed upon this inexperienced impressionability.[33]

Her words were therefore designed precisely to undermine Coleridge's paternalistic polemic, appealing specifically to a calculus of humanity and to a female vulnerability that she accused Coleridge of exploiting. She wrote of her long-felt 'need of a Society such as I have now joined, to defend the eminent scientists and surgeons who devote their lives to the alleviation of human suffering, from the unwarrantable attacks made upon their humanity by your Society'. She accused Coleridge and his society of promoting 'sensational' literature and imagery, which 'work on the sympathies of the public, – and especially on the feelings of the female sex – and you thus keep alive an agitation which is mainly based on ignorance of facts, and maintained by persistent misrepresentation'. It was, without question, a battle for the sentiments of the public, based on the manipulation of their sympathies. Antivivisectionist manipulation was, in this view, corrupt, whereas the RDS was said to have evidence and a true humanitarian purpose on its side. Its truths were difficult for an uneducated sentimentalism to grasp, whereas antivivisectionist propaganda worked precisely to amplify such affective ignorance. Ultimately, Montrose alluded to the 'immense importance of such experiments to the welfare of mankind; and the great saving of human life which is already due to them' and she hoped that the RDS would 'enlighten the public' as to the 'direct advantage to humanity derived from physiological research'.[34]

The argument was standard enough. It was well-rehearsed rhetoric: a script. It was characteristic of RDS literature, to be sure, and recapitulated a position maintained principally by physiologists since the 1870s. The argument had been effective from that date, especially in terms of formal protection of medical research from antivivisectionist inroads. In the years immediately following the Brown Dog Affair, however, the perceived need to capture the support of the public (or, at least, those parts of the public deemed to be worth counting) was greater than ever. The source of the words therefore became as important as their content. Not only did society women speak with a perceived first-hand knowledge or lived experience of refined sensibility, they also could speak, as Montrose did, with knowledge of the vulnerability of such sensibility in

---

[33] 'Research Defence Society', compilation of correspondence in *The Times*, to which added Duchess of Montrose to Stephen Coleridge, 28 December 1908, RDS Occasional Publications and Printed Papers, SA/RDS/G/1/10: Box 13, Wellcome Library, London.

[34] 'Research Defence Society', compilation of correspondence in *The Times*, to which added Duchess of Montrose to Stephen Coleridge, 28 December 1908, 6–7, RDS Occasional Publications and Printed Papers, SA/RDS/G/1/10: Box 13, Wellcome Library, London.

the inexperienced and uneducated, and the risk of its corruption by unscrupulous and misinformed powerful men.

In this case, the RDS received the additional support of an editorial in *The Times* that precisely echoed Montrose's letter to Coleridge. 'The movement towards humane treatment of animals, and careful avoidance of the infliction upon them of needless suffering, is, in itself, entirely admirable. But when people allow that excellent impulse to dominate them, to become a fixed idea, and to render them incapable of giving their due place to other things equally admirable and equally noble, humanitarian sentiment becomes a pernicious sentimentalism.' Coleridge, written off as a 'pertinacious and not too scrupulous controversialist', was one of many for whom a 'passionate sympathy with animals ... is shown by, among other things, the extraordinary caprice with which that sympathy is bestowed'.[35]

Here, then, were two humanitarian scripts running on a collision course. The impact of one on the other would reveal the resolution of one form of sympathy into viciousness and risk the loss of the substantial sympathy that activated medical research, to the detriment of humanity itself. Again, there was nothing particularly new about this formulation. It was the stock position of medical research and its scientific supporters. The active recruitment and employment of society women and other eminent lay figures to promote it was, however, an innovative turn.

Eminent Laymen

If a lady counted three, a cleric counted four. At a meeting of the Cambridge branch of the RDS in March 1910, chaired by George Darwin (1845–1912) (could there be a more powerful symbol of the Darwinian roots of opposition to antivivisection?), the Bishop of Ely, Frederic Chase (1853–1925), gave a pointedly dispassionate speech in favour of animal research in which he explicitly set out to 'deal with the appeal to emotion'. His view, which he arrived at explicitly as a thinking layman, was that the right of dominion over animals, coupled with an intent to reduce the suffering of humans, made animal experimentation a 'duty'. But, he lamented, it was 'just at this point ... that emotion comes in, the emotion of pity'. If the 'attention' were fixed on animal suffering, it would be possible to 'decide the whole controversy on the simple ground of that appeal to emotion', he said. In other words, emotion got in the way of rational and detached inquiry and therefore to a proper understanding of the relative painlessness of

---

[35] 'Research Defence Society', compilation of correspondence in *The Times*, to which added Duchess of Montrose to Stephen Coleridge, 28 December 1908, 7, RDS Occasional Publications and Printed Papers, SA/RDS/G/1/10: Box 13, Wellcome Library, London.

experimental research. Yet despite a desire to bracket emotion, this rational view still involved a calculus of suffering, wherein human suffering was weighed in the balance of animal suffering, and the scale of each compared. This was not activated by a sense of pity but by 'the sense of responsibility' that comes with true research and with an appreciation of the challenge of 'lessening ... the whole sum of the suffering which is in the world'.[36]

Chase's speech followed another by Cromer, the RDS President, giving the whole affair the credibility of conservative lay opinion. This was mirrored by the Oxford Branch of the RDS, which was predicated on attracting such support. The inimitable William Archibald Spooner (1844–1930), Warden of (cue knowledge) New College, Oxford, 'made a strong appeal to laymen to support the work of the Society' in the branch's inaugural public meeting in October 1910.[37] Lord Cromer was again in attendance, and the branch's president was the unimpeachable figure of William Osler. Osler could hardly be classed a layman, given his fame as a physician, but he was no experimenter himself. He had, however, spent his whole career defending medical science. Osler had been a star witness before the second Royal Commission, speaking with authority about the overwhelming human benefit of experimental insight – the instinct to follow certain courses according to the experience of animal experimentation – that had wrought great leaps in knowledge in the transmission of, for example, malaria and yellow fever. Osler had been asked about the experience of American medical science, untrammelled by legislation, in comparison to the English case. His answer was characteristic of what would become the core messaging of the RDS, characterized by a barely concealed restraint, and indicative of a core affective quality that defined experimental practice and practitioners. Osler spoke not as a practitioner himself, but as man of standing who had personal knowledge of men he felt impugned by the English public:

Personally, I feel that the matter could be left safely in the hands of the men who are in charge of the physiological laboratories and the scientific men of this country. I feel, of course, rather strongly; I would not like, perhaps, to express my feelings as strongly as they exist on what I regard has been in some ways a standing insult to the humanity of these men. They have been hounded by a great section of the public in a way that I think is disgraceful to the English people. These are men who have lived lives of devotion and self-sacrifice, and belonging to a group of men whose service to humanity has been so incalculable that they ought not to be treated in the way they have been.... I know these men;

[36] The Bishop of Ely, *Humanity and Science* (London: Research Defence Society, 1910), SA/RDS/G/1/18, Wellcome Library, London.
[37] RDS Oxford Branch Minutes of 24 October 1910, Oxford Branch Minute Book, 12, SA/RDS/C/17: Box 6, Wellcome Library, London.

they are just as humane as any other men; and to place these vexatious restrictions upon them is an insult, I think.[38]

It should be no wonder that Osler headed the initiative to set up a branch of the RDS in Oxford. When he spoke on the stage at the group's inaugural meeting, behind him in silent support sat Stephen Paget, RDS Honorary Secretary and the Lord Bishop of Oxford. His Grace happened to be Francis Paget (1851–1911), Stephen's brother. The affinity between men of the high church and men of science should not be underestimated. The success of the RDS was largely garnered through . personal connections that already existed. If the alignment of lay society and the scientific community seems surprising on the face of it, small incidental genealogical facts such as this ought to prove telling. They are emblematic of the extent to which men of science had become entrenched at the vanguard of public influence and value, and of the fine line between lives that were steered into the paths of religion and research. New priesthood and old shared the platform. The problem that Stephen Paget recognized, and that defined the RDS, was that the neophytes could not command the same respect in the court of public opinion as could their brothers in the church. They were therefore put to service as mouthpieces and, as in this case, physical presences of support.

All of this is characteristic of a society, branching out across the country, which aimed to finesse an association with scientists and doctors into a vindication of their practices, without having constantly to hear from the scientists themselves. In Birmingham, for example, the committee formally considered strategies of 'approaching the laity', which resulted in public meetings, pamphleteering, newspaper advertisements and the writing of circular letters. In the Kensington branch, thousands of invitations were distributed to targeted members of polite society to come and hear public lectures in support of animal experimentation. At one such meeting in June 1910, a packed Town Hall crowd of 400 came to hear Stephen Paget lecture on 'What we owe to experiments on animals', but it was the speech of Sir David Gill (1843–1914), committee member of the Kensington branch of the RDS and chair of the public meeting, that made the press.

Gill was just the sort of respectable layman the RDS hoped to find. As a celebrated astronomer, already well into his sixties, Gill carried with him the respect accorded to a scientific mind, though he had no obvious vested interest in medicine or medical research. He was the kind of figure who exuded public trustworthiness. Gill said that 'it should hardly be necessary to protest so strongly that it was essential to inquire into

---

[38] UK Parliament, Appendix to the Fourth Report of the Commissioners, C. 3955 (1908), 161.

scientific truth, more particularly when that truth was concerned with the saving of human life and the alleviation of human suffering; and yet there were those possessed of a curious idea that a scientific man, at least in the department of medicine, was a species of human fiend'. So far, so orthodox. But then he rhetorically appealed to what he thought was a natural alignment of femininity and medical science: 'Let any mother of a child afflicted with an incipient attack of diphtheria ask how many guinea pigs she would give for the life of her child', he said, to which a woman's voice answered loudly 'None'. Here, in a public meeting, populated principally by a lay crowd, was the kind of front-line exchange that was characteristic of what happened when pro- and antivivisection camps actually engaged in person. It was hardly an intellectual exchange. Gill sought clarification: had a lady really said 'none'? 'Not one', came the reply. Gill responded dismissively: 'That is a very fair example of the common-sense of the people who oppose scientific research. If that is humanity, God help humanity!' Press reports note that Gill was met with cheers and applause, as well as a few hisses from the ranks of hecklers.

Narratives such as this have to be read for what they represent, rather than for anything particular about what was said. Gill's exclamation about 'humanity' exactly represented the core argument of medical science from the previous thirty years. It signifies the transition of a scientific argument into a vernacular idiom. It did not need elaboration or substantiation, at least not from Gill (Paget, as the voice of the parent society, provided this). The mere repetition of the slogan, given the natural authority of the source, was sufficient. It was met with cheers and applause, the sonorous signs of civilization, as well as 'hisses' from the antis. Hissing painted the opponents of experimental research as themselves animalistic, unworthy of civilized company and unfit for a civilized space. The press reports therefore did the work of the RDS beautifully. The clippings were proudly pasted into the Kensington branch minute book.[39]

RDS activity in its early years must be viewed as an alignment of moral and medical progressivism on the one hand, and class paternalism, even conservatism, on the other, with a distinctly gendered tone. In fact, it would be better to say that the defence of experimental medicine was a direct expression of class paternalism, since it assumed the enemies of medical science to be those of low social status, low or no education and emotional primitiveness. Opponents of vivisection literally did not know what was

---

[39] The reports were remarkably consistent in their description of the event. The minute book includes clippings from the *Daily Mail*, *Daily News*, *Morning Post*, *Standard*, and one more unidentified report. RDS Kensington Branch minute book, SA/RDS/C/16: Box 6, pasted after the minute for 27 May 1910, Wellcome Library, London.

good for them and they were too easily swayed by salacious arguments and provocative imagery. This put 'education' at the heart of RDS activity, but this category must be construed both positively and negatively. Yes, there were significant efforts to elaborate and disseminate the medical and public-health benefits of medical experimentation, but there were equal efforts to persuade the public of both the unscrupulous nature of antivivisectionism and of the moral attitude of medical research. This latter thread depended enormously upon the RDS association with prominent society figures who were not directly connected to science. As the Birmingham branch of the RDS claimed in a release placed in the *Birmingham Gazette and Express* in January 1910, among the RDS membership were 'many distinguished men and women, whose names alone are a warranty for the goodness of its cause'. It was almost as if the message was unnecessary, given the messengers. That message, for what it was worth, was relayed by RDS President, Lord Cromer, whose note was included in the Birmingham press release: 'it is … necessary to keep constantly before the eyes of the general public the fact that the bacteriologist, whose researches tend to prolong life and mitigate suffering, and not the antivivisectionist, is the true friend of humanity'. While Professor R. F. C. Leith (d. 1936), the Birmingham branch society chair, understood the RDS to be a 'great educational movement' to support 'efforts which are being made to combat disease and its offspring, disablement and death', he nevertheless paused to point out that 'ladies are particularly welcome' to subscribe.[40]

It would be all too easy to characterize the RDS as a pro-scientific research pressure group, but I think this misses the point. The RDS understood scientific research to be a particular expression of civilizational status and its activity was therefore geared towards safeguarding a particular valuation of society. Both its ends and its means were therefore social. While medical experimentation was the primary beneficiary of the RDS's particular efforts, the broader aim was conservative. It should not be a surprise that the RDS was heir to the evolutionary argument about a higher form of sympathy or humanity that could be dispensed via the knowledge gained in the laboratory. That argument was formed at the cutting edge, literally, of science, but had depended on gentlemanliness and reputation, on the paternalism of independent wealth in support of a rapidly professionalizing science. In the years before the First World War, the success of that argument can be measured by the extent to which it had willingly been co-opted by social elites. If Darwin had seen himself as an evolutionary saltation – a great adaptive leap defined by intellectual insight and emotional

---

[40] *Birmingham Gazette and Express*, 27 January 1910. Cutting pasted into RDS Birmingham Branch minute book, 33, SA/RDS/C/15: Box 6, Wellcome Library, London.

detachment – he, and notable followers such as Galton, had made his appeals as a part of, even as a justification of, the social status quo. It was much easier for social elites to fasten themselves to this vision than to entertain the radical levelling of a civilizational meritocracy à la Huxley. Medical science had fashioned itself, from the 1870s, as a secular religion, an elite defined by its social knowledge, and most moderately as a professional influence for the good of society at large. It is unsurprising that progressive members of the aristocracy who could tell which way the wind was blowing, as well as ambitious members of the rising middle classes, would flock to the cause.

It must be remembered, however, that the RDS did have instrumental ends in mind. Paget was policing public discourse, answering antivivisectionist rhetoric wherever it cropped up. He kept the medical humanitarian message alive and fresh in the minds of polite society, and worked upon the hearts of 'the masses'. The RDS did not hope to win over the ranks of the working classes through rational argument, but through the building of trust in medicine, and sowing the seeds of mistrust in antivivisection. Paget and his allies did not expect everyone to be able to extol the virtues of animal experimentation, but they did hope that they could induce people to *feel* that the RDS brand of humanity was the right brand. As Cromer wrote in the introductory essay to a volume summarizing the testimony of scientists in favour of vivisection before the Royal Commission, true humanity was at stake. He felt 'that they were, under circumstances which rendered them peculiarly liable to misrepresentation, fighting a cause in which not only the whole human race, but also the brute creation, were deeply interested'. He wrote that 'it was not merely unjust, but also unwise, that the medical profession should be allowed to stand alone in the defence of a noble cause.[41] A noble cause required not merely technical expertise and specialist qualifications, but noble allies. The simple association of the expert word with such societal figures would, so it was thought, serve to amplify the truth, or at least gild it. The reduction of the rationale of medical humanitarianism to its most essential slogans, delivered via figures assumed to be implicitly trustworthy – ladies, churchmen, gentlemen – was heart work. It was an attempt to alter the emotional register and reception of experimentation, to fundamentally transform the immediate visceral reaction to the word or image of vivisection.

---

[41] Lord Cromer, 'Introduction', in Paget, *For and Against Experiments*, xii.

Experiment and the Crown

Until 1913, experimental medicine had been an essentially private affair. The government, under the auspices of the Local Government Board, could sponsor research if it deemed it necessary, and John Simon had been a great friend of the physiological community in particular. But the history of animal experimentation until 1913 was predominantly a story of private funding for private initiatives, with the defence of experimental practices on humanitarian and knowledge-production grounds coming from the medical community and its supporters on their own initiative. The government, as we have seen, was limited to a regulatory role, which was in turn tendered out to the medical community. All of this would change with the foundation of the Medical Research Committee (MRC; later, the Medical Research Council) in 1913. Its emergence capped a generation of strategic efforts on the part of the medical community to gain acceptance and institutionalization for experimental research.

All the while, the AAMR continued to be the government's de facto administrator of applications for licences under the 1876 Act. This continued until 1913 when, on the basis of the second Royal Commission's report, a new arrangement was put in place to make sure that there could no longer be any direct conflict of interest in the vetting of applications. While this might have introduced a new inconvenience for medical scientists, the reality was that the government had become experimental research's chief sponsor, and its increasing interest in public health was only increasing its investment in experimental techniques. The story of this development is, in some ways, separate from long-standing questions regarding the defence of experimental medicine, but this thread would become entangled with the other.

In 1901, the government had sponsored a Royal Commission on Tuberculosis, specifically to investigate its causes, the connections between human and animal varieties, and the means of its transmission. The appointed Commissioners, chaired by Michael Foster, who had been at the forefront of work using experimental animals for a generation, took a radical approach to their duty, by eschewing the usual course of calling expert witnesses and instead setting about an entirely experimental enquiry. It would take ten years. In those ten years, the Crown effectively paid for a programme of experimental research on living animals – bovines, goats, pigs, chimpanzees, monkeys, lemurs, dogs, cats, mongoose, hedgehogs, rabbits, guinea pigs, rats and mice – picking up a thread of concern that had especially occupied medical scientists for a generation and making it a direct concern of government.[42] The final cost of the Commission was £75 645.[43] The questions set to the Commissioners implied an experimental course of action. The entire series of reports and appendices were experimental in nature. And the conclusions were suggestive of further experimentation.

In its coverage of the Final Report of the Commission, the *Lancet* was laudatory of the spirit of strict experimental professionalism that had defined the work of the Commissioners, lamenting the fact that 'the Commission is not to be organised into a permanent bureau'.[44] While there was a hiatus, the sentiment was also felt at the level of government.

Such was the degree of concern, dovetailing with new initiatives to shore up the health of the populace, and in the competitive spirit of matching the industrial and civilizing progress of Germany, that the tuberculosis issue became an integral part of the National Insurance Act of 1911. Under a clause having specifically to do with administering sanatorium benefits for 'insured persons suffering from tuberculosis or *any other such disease* [emphasis mine]', the Act made provision of one penny per insured person for research. The ambiguity of focus introduced by the clause came with enormous possibilities for the future of experimental medicine.[45] While historiographical focus has largely been on the tensions caused by the Act among the medical community, concerning doctors' pay and responsibilities under it, the research clause was never anything but a coup for the experimental establishment.

This clause was in the original Bill, introduced by David Lloyd George (1863–1945) in May 1911, and it remained there, essentially unamended, through to its Royal Ascent. Lloyd George himself wondered at the almost astonishing lack of attention given to this clause, both in the House and in the Press, perhaps because it so pointedly made medical research a government responsibility. Arthur Balfour (1848–1930) quizzed him, in an early debate on the Bill, about the need for scientific research, noting that 'it is not really possible to waste money if you devote it judiciously to scientific, medical investigations into the causes and cure of the disease'. 'Let us take care', he said, 'that we do not spend too much of our money on inanimate structures [sanatoria] ... and that we spend a little more in carrying out those further schemes of research and investigation on which

[42] UK Parliament, Final Report of the Royal Commission Appointed to Inquire into the Relation of Human and Animal Tuberculosis, C. 5761 (1911).

[43] John Francis, 'The Work of the British Royal Commission on Tuberculosis, 1901–1911', *Tubercle*, 40 (1959): 128.

[44] 'The Royal Commission on Human and Bovine Tuberculosis', *The Lancet*, 15 July 1911, 167.

[45] 1 & 2 geo. 5. Ch. 55 (1911), 16.1.a.

the real progress of the race in these medical matters most assuredly rests'.[46] Lloyd George assured him that the government would make 'a contribution, under proper scientific direction, which will enable us to arrive at something sooner or later which will enable us effectively to stamp out this terrible disease … we are making a contribution towards Scientific Research'.[47] It must have been a rare occurrence indeed to find agreement across the aisle in the Parliament of 1911. It suggests that the both sides of the House were willing to entertain medical research as the province of the Crown in the name of public health. The accord would effectively mute opposition.

In response to the passing of the National Insurance Act, the Local Government Board appointed a Departmental Committee to report on what the government's general policy might be towards tuberculosis, which centred heavily on the question of future medical research, and what to do with the available funds generated by the Act. Such a committee was implied under clause 8.1.b of the Act, which pertained to the range of diseases that the Act would serve. While tuberculosis was the only disease specifically mentioned, it was clear in the wording of the Act that it would not be the sole remit of it. Attention to this clause has been largely missed in research into the origins of the MRC, because the clause specific to research was contained in 16.2.b of the Act. Yet the whole of clause 16 referred to 'tuberculosis or any other such disease as aforesaid', and this fore-saying was found in clause 8. Here it was stated that 'treatment in sanatoria or other institutions or other wise' could be granted when 'suffering from tuberculosis, or such other diseases as the Local Government Board with the approval of the Treasury may appoint'. This foreshadowed clause 16, which provided for the financing of such treatment and was inclusive of research.[48] While scholars have wondered what Lloyd George intended by allowing funds for research – whether research on tuberculosis alone, or a broader agenda – it is clear in the discussion of clause 8 that, while tuberculosis loomed largest in the minds of the drafters of the Bill, other diseases were always in mind. Surprisingly, the terms of what was specifically meant by 'other diseases', or how the Local Government Board might 'appoint' them, was not debated in committee during the passage of the National Insurance Bill, despite an amendment on this clause tabled by Austen Chamberlain (1863–1937).[49]

Austen Chamberlain's criticism of clause 8.1.b of the Bill, which he proposed to leave out, concerned the 'propriety of this special treatment of the disease of tuberculosis', since the 'very peculiar treatment of this

[46] *Hansard*, fifth series, 25, col. 2065, 17 May 1911.
[47] *Hansard*, fifth series, 25, cols. 2066–8, 17 May 1911   [48] 1 & 2 geo. 5. Ch. 55 (1911).
[49] *Hansard*, fifth series, 28, col. 385, 12 July 1911.

one disease is, for good or evil . . . an excrescence on the general scheme of the Bill'. He pointed out that the Bill did not 'make special provision in this way for the treatment of any other disease', and said, 'I do not know why'.[50] This, it seems to me, was a flawed reading of the Bill, which contained, even at the draft stage, the phrase 'such other diseases'. What is extraordinary about the very long debate that followed was the singular focus on tuberculosis, and the absolute failure of anybody, including Lloyd George, to point out Austen Chamberlain's mistaken reading. Contained in this debate is the only substantial discussion of the importance of research, upon which there was almost complete agreement. Only George Barnes, one of the first Labour MPs in Scotland, sounded a note of alarm: 'I am not going to say anything against scientific research, but I think it is something which ought to be carefully watched, and if we are going to have scientific research I want it to be safeguarded. I hope we shall not torture any more poor dumb animals for the purpose of scientific research'.[51] His concern went unremarked and unanswered in the debate. Austen Chamberlain withdrew his amendment, based on Lloyd George's reply about the usefulness of sanatoria, and the clause found its way unaltered into the Act.

Historians of the MRC, specifically Landsborough Thomson and Linda Bryder, made no headway in determining why Lloyd George inserted this broad ambiguity about the potential scope of research and of the definition of 'disease'.[52] Bryder thought it 'of little consequence who was responsible for proposing the clause on research for the Act', because she was not interested in its past, but in the 'subsequent career of the clause in the hands of the Departmental Committee on Tuberculosis'.[53] But it strikes me that both the vague definition of the diseases to be treated under the terms of the National Insurance Act and the proposal to fund medical research in this broad category of 'disease' were themselves of significant moment for a generation-long campaign of the medical establishment to safeguard the profession. It is not, then, a question of which individual was responsible for the insertion of the research clause. Rather, the presence of that clause might itself be seen as the effect of the general pressure brought to bear on government concerning the value and utility

[50] *Hansard*, fifth series, 28, col. 385, 12 July 1911.
[51] *Hansard*, fifth series, 28, col. 417, 12 July 1911.
[52] A. Landsborough Thomson, 'Origin of the British Legislative Provision for Medical Research', *Journal of Social Policy*, 2 (1973): 41–54; Linda Bryder, 'Tuberculosis and the MRC', in *Historical Perspectives on the Role of the MRC: Essays in the History of the Medical Research Council of the United Kingdom and Its Predecessor, the Medical Research Committee, 1913–1953*, ed. Joan Austoker and Linda Bryder (Oxford: Oxford University Press, 1989), 1–5.
[53] Bryder, 'Tuberculosis and the MRC', 3.

of medical research.[54] The timing of it is remarkable. While the Royal Commission on Vivisection would not issue its final report until 1912, its proceedings were well enough known for the government to be able to foresee a change in the way that experimental research would be administered, and the overwhelming weight of expert testimony continued to be in favour of animal experimentation on humanitarian grounds. The final report of the Royal Commission on Tuberculosis was issued in the middle of the debates of the National Insurance Bill, and was roundly celebrated throughout Parliament as being of immense value. Vivisection had, essentially, been vindicated twice. The government could, for the first time, consider sponsoring medical research involving animals without moral compunction. The human cost of not doing so, according to the parliamentary debates, was simply too awful to entertain.

The funds ultimately made available for research were estimated to be in the order of £57 000 annually.[55] Leaving aside the Royal Commission on Tuberculosis, which was not necessarily intended as direct government funding of medical research, this represented a massive paradigm shift in government policy vis-à-vis experiment. It would effectively make the matter of defence, on ethical and humanitarian grounds, an issue of the Crown. As the Departmental Committee organized to work out how to spend the

[54] Responsibility for the research clause may well lie with Lloyd George himself. A great deal of speculation has been carried out to attribute credit for this to Christopher Addison (1869–1951). Doubtless, Addison did serve as the major go-between for Lloyd George and the BMA as the Bill was hashed out, but Addison himself denied having initiated the research clause and, even though some scholars have pointed out that Lloyd George said, in 1914, that Addison was 'mainly responsible for committing the Government to the very important question of medical research work', they fail to point out that Addison, on the same occasion, told the medical community that 'the medical profession owed a debt of gratitude to Mr. Lloyd George for the establishment of the scheme of medical research'. 'Dinner to the Dr. Christopher Addison, M.P.', *Lancet*, 14 February 1914, 483. Cf. Frank Honigsbaum, 'Christopher Addison: A Realist in Pursuit of Dreams', in *Doctors, Politics and Society: Historical Essays*, ed. Dorothy Porter and Roy Porter (Amsterdam: Rodopi, 1993), 230–31; K. Morgan, 'Addison, Christopher, First Viscount Addison (1869–1951), Politician', in *Oxford Dictionary of National Biography*; Landsborough Thomson, 'Origin and Development', 1290; Bryder, 'Tuberculosis and the MRC', 3; Harvey Cushing, *The Life of Sir William Osler* (Oxford, 1940), ii, 1151n1. There is evidence in Addison's papers at the Bodleian Library that he was well connected with the specific aims and agenda of the RDS, well before his involvement in the NI Bill, and this may well be the most significant factor in attributing the clause in the NI Bill to him. But he does not appear to have acted as explicitly as an agent for the RDS, suggesting rather that RDS arguments had been generally adopted by this time among the medical establishment. Safeguarding the funding and the rationale for medical research was, by 1911, both an obvious and an *essential* thing to do, from the point of view of the vast majority of medical scientists and doctors. Addison happened to be best placed to carry this out. See Addison Papers, Bodleian Library, Oxford, MS. Addison dep. c. 8, file *d*, fols 265–292.

[55] UK Parliament, Final Report of the Departmental Committee on Tuberculosis, C. 6641 (1913), vol. 1, 13.

money itself reported, the 'provision marks a most important development in the attitude of the State towards scientific research into the causes, treatment and prevention of disease'.[56] Crucially, despite the Committee's express purpose of reporting on tuberculosis, they mirrored the National Insurance Act's broad terms about the scope of any 'research' to which public funds might be applied. While they anticipated that 'the moneys will be applied mainly to research in connection with tuberculosis and its allied problems', they nevertheless entertained the 'possibility of extension of research to other diseases' and that whatever 'machinery' was to be established ought to 'facilitate such an extension'.[57] This position had been arrived at via the collection of expert testimony, including from overseas, and on the basis of legal advice.[58]

It was in these terms that the Committee recommended the foundation of a permanent body of paid 'experts' who could determine precisely how the NI money should be spent. This was the basis for the foundation of the Medical Research Committee, which began its business in July 1913.[59] Its first Committee included important figures from the Departmental Committee on Tuberculosis, Waldorf Astor (1879–1952), son of the American owner of the *Observer* and *Pall Mall Gazette*, and Christopher Addison, by then the medical profession's most important ally in Westminster. And it was chaired by Fletcher Moulton, whose friendliness to the cause of experimental medicine has already been substantially shown. The MRC thus had cross-bench political backing as well as the strings of public opinion at its disposal (Astor would himself come into possession of his father's newspapers in 1914, and had been the instigator of the *Observer* purchase in 1911).[60] For the medical-scientific community, it was a great boon: an epoch-defining shift in government policy, yes, but also a transformative cultural moment for the place of scientific research in public life. For the first time, medical scientists would become official employees of the state, with state sanction for their research.

At a dinner meeting prior to the MRC's first official Committee meeting, held at Fletcher Moulton's house, the members-to-be were introduced to the Chair of the Commission to implement the National

[56] UK Parliament, Final Report of the Departmental Committee on Tuberculosis, C. 6641 (1913), vol. 1, 13.
[57] UK Parliament, Final Report of the Departmental Committee on Tuberculosis, C. 6641 (1913), 1:14.
[58] Bryder, 'Tuberculosis and the MRC', 4–5. Bryder specifically mentions the input of Simon Flexner.
[59] MRC Minute of 24 July 1913, Minutes of the Meetings of the Medical Research Committee, 1913, 1914, FD 6/1, National Archives, London.
[60] Alfred M. Gollin, *The Observer and J. L. Garvin, 1908–1914* (London: Oxford University Press, 1960), 300–303.

Insurance Act, Robert Morant (1863–1920). He told them of the money available per annum, and noted that 'it was hoped that the money would not be employed simply to endow or bolster up institutions or individuals'. In short, the government wanted a new, national effort at medical research. Moulton then asked the members to suggest subjects 'most suitable for investigation' and found, in an open question-and-answer session, that 'our field was as wide as we chose to make it, Tuberculosis being merely *one* of the first subjects which would engage us'.[61] Thus, even before its formal beginning, the MRC had effectively abandoned the singular focus on tuberculosis that had dominated political debate, and instead pursued an agenda that accorded not only with the letter of the law, but with the prevailing spirit of knowledge production within the experimental-medicine community. The MRC would encapsulate the whole argument and ethos of the provivisection position, and necessarily so. For while the research agenda was wide open, all the legal advice had suggested that any research had to be connected to 'disease to which insured persons may be liable' and 'as bore some definite relation to improvement in the methods of prevention and treatment of disease'.[62] Thus, MRC experimental endeavours were to be humanitarian by definition, according to the government legal advice and the enshrined in law. It was, therefore, not merely a national institutionalization of research, but an institutionalization of the rationale of research and an endorsement of its fundamentally humanitarian purpose. This lent a structural power to the basic position of medical scientists that was hitherto unknown.

The full implications of the establishment of the MRC were quickly realized. Not only did the first Committee understand its remit to go far beyond the question of tuberculosis, it also understood the importance of establishing an institution of state-run medical research. Very quickly, it devised a National Institute for Medical Research at Hampstead, at the site vacated by the Mount Vernon Hospital and it set about establishing departments, of bacteriology, pharmacology and biochemistry, applied physiology and statistics, with senior figures hired to head them.[63] It was clear from the start that work 'must be done on animals' and a target list of diseases and disease problems was drawn up, including 'disease "carriers"', meningitis, polio, syphilis, measles, whooping cough, scarlet fever, occupational

---

[61] Papers of Sir William Leishman, bound into a single volume, 176, 'Medical Research Committee, Dinner Meeting at L M's', RAMC/563: Box 124, Wellcome Library, London.

[62] Bryder, 'Tuberculosis and the MRC', 4–5.

[63] MRC Minute of 19 March 1914, Minutes of the Meetings of the Medical Research Committee, 1913, 1914, FD 6/1, National Archives, London.

diseases, colour blindness, food adulterations and standards of purity and sociological problems (housing, ventilation, child labour, school hygiene).[64]

The First World War is a breaking point in this narrative, changing the context in which medical-scientific experimentation was received. As with so many other fringe political issues, antivivisection was given far less oxygen at a time of national emergency. Yet is important to stress that these key events in the two years prior to the outbreak of war had effectively sealed a long-term victory for medical experimentation. Any rhetorical arguments from the antivivisection camp would now have to uproot not just the principles and justifications for experimentation put forward by scientists and their lay allies, but to uproot experimentation as a well-funded activity of the Crown, replete with institutions and a consensus of implicit political support.

Shop Talk

'Lizzie' Lind af Hageby, the arch antivivisectionist, opened a shop on Piccadilly in London from which she sold and distributed antivivisectionist literature. The shop right next door was leased by the RDS, which remained, by the outbreak of war, the principal strategic institution of the medical establishment and of its public supporters for the protection and promotion of medical-scientific research using living animals (Figure 4.2). The RDS had its own literature to distribute. The RDS hired a man to stand outside their 'shop' to hand-out leaflets and to distract any many members of the public who were attracted to Lind af Hageby's shop. Lind af Hageby hired a man in turn. The two men, apparently, got along. Neither, as far as the record shows, had any personal interest in the respective causes. They were essentially bouncers for public hearts.

It is an eccentric scene: a Piccadilly circus. The RDS were obviously threatened by the activities of Lind af Hageby and had identified her London shop as the epicentre of antivivisection in England. For a cause that is best known for its pamphleteering and rhetoric, it is a curio to think of it having a physical location, a shop window, a saleswoman, a doorman.[65] It is equally quirky to think of the medical establishment renting a shop in order to mirror this physical presence, as if the battle for public opinion could be won by the best window display. Lind af Hageby testified that she had felt compelled to hire her own doorman

---

[64] Papers of Sir William Leishman, bound into a single volume, 179, '2nd Meeting', RAMC/563: Box 124, Wellcome Library, London.

[65] There were a number of such shops throughout the country, run by Frances Power Cobbe's British Union for the Abolition of Vivisection. See Bates, *Anti-Vivisection and the Profession of Medicine*, 140.

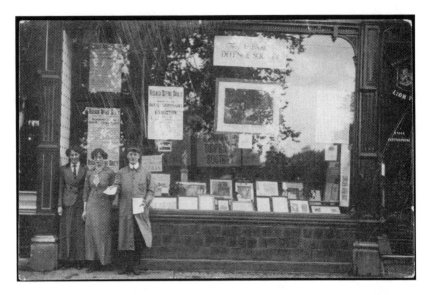

Figure 4.2 Research Defence Society Shop, Piccadilly. Wellcome Library, London. Attribution 4.0 International (CC BY 4.0).

because the arm of the RDS doorman had waved in front of her shop, beckoning 'customers' away from her window. This, she felt, was a transgression of space. The emissary of vivisection had crossed the line projecting forward from the boundary of her premises and thereby contaminated a space that she had designated as antivivisection space. She remonstrated with the man, to no effect, and thereafter employed her own to police the line and disseminate the message. The two men must have made an odd couple.[66]

All of this seems prosaic, parochial or trivial. It is not. In 1913, Lind af Hageby sued Caleb Saleeby (1878–1940), the physician and eugenics popularizer, for libel. Also included in the suit were the *Pall Mall Gazette* and its owner, William Waldorf Astor (1848–1919). It is, justifiably, a famous trial, which Lind af Hageby lost. Saleeby had accused her of running 'a systematic campaign of falsehood' in her antivivisection activities.[67] In this point, he was vindicated. But the trial is remembered principally because Lind af Hageby represented herself, at a time when women were barred from practising law. Her

[66] In the High Court of Justice Kings Bench Division, Before: Mr Justice Bucknill and a Special Jury, Lind-af-Hageby v Astor & Others, Third Day, Thursday, 3 April 1913, 3–4, 41, GC/89/3, Wellcome Library, London.
[67] C. W. Saleeby, 'The House of Life. The Waste of Mercy', *Pall Mall Gazette*, 7 May 1912.

oratory, testimony, cross-examinations and even-tempered carriage were celebrated as a milestone for the cause of women in public life. The specifics of her case have become relatively unimportant compared with its contribution to narrative accounts of the emancipation of women.

Re-visiting the case and, without wishing to diminish Lind af Hageby's performance, re-reading it for what it says about the character of the opposition she faced, one is struck by the sense of what is at stake here: civilization itself. One particular strand of the libel trial concerned a line in Saleeby's *Pall Mall Gazette* piece that claimed Lind af Hageby had made Piccadilly in London 'almost impassable for decent people'.[68] Here is the nub of the argument and its magnitude. Once Saleeby sounded off in the *Gazette*, then Piccadilly was everywhere. Lind af Hageby's shop was no longer just a physical space with fronting to the street. It became a shop in the minds and imaginations of anybody who read Saleeby's piece. All of those readers, one might suppose, would have considered themselves 'decent people'. The prospect of a space in the metropolis that was unfit for them was, on principle, to be abhorred. Lind af Hageby, in her libel suit, made the claim that it was the RDS who were making the street unfit for passers-by. She did not have the better of the argument. Even across the Atlantic, the medical establishment watched Lind af Hageby's suit with interest, having had direct experience with her brand of antivivisection. Simon Flexner, director of the Rockefeller Institute for Medical Research (about which much more in the following chapter), wrote to Paget after Lind af Hageby's loss, declaring: 'We are all rejoiced over the result of the damage suit brought by Miss Hageby and are hoping that it may abate somewhat your disturbing antivivisection troubles'.[69]

Here then, in a spat about the sale of pamphlets in the heart of the capital, was the core of the establishment strategy against antivivisection: to call it out as anti-civilization and anti-progress. Antivivisection was branded anti-intellectual in its refusal to acknowledge the well-advertised benefits of animal research. And antivivisectionists like Lind af Hageby could hardly claim ignorance of these arguments. They emanated from the shop next door.

The constellation of forces arrayed against Lind af Hageby was, perhaps, unbeatable. Antivivisection had made no real headway in the second Royal Commission, the findings of which had in any case been superseded by the National Insurance Act and the creation of the MRC. Once the Crown was in the business of vivisection, there was little

---

[68] Saleeby, 'The House of Life. The Waste of Mercy'.
[69] Flexner to Paget, 4 June 1913, Flexner Paget correspondence, Reel 86, FA746, Series 1 Simon Flexner Paper; Subseries 1.2 Rockefeller Institute for Medical Research, Simon Flexner Papers (American Philosophical Society), RAC.

hope for its detractors. This was all the more the case because of the overlap of interests of the Astor family. With one Astor steering medical research under the auspices of a publicly funded institution, and another running one of the principal public lines of defence in the *Pall Mall Gazette*, medical science had successfully developed and safeguarded its experimental methods.

The AAMR, having lost its pseudo-official function in 1913, effectively lost its purpose. It could still advise applicants for licences, but it could no longer advocate on behalf of those applicants with the Home Office. Stephen Paget, having made a success of his move to the RDS, could suggest by 1916 that the AAMR might be amalgamated with his society. The RDS could provide the advisory function, and the establishment could pay one subscription instead of two.[70] The offer was repeated in early 1917 and acceded to. The AAMR at that point had 114 members and £280 in the bank.[71] The disappearance of the AAMR was a sign of its astonishing success over thirty-five years. When the RDS reported its work to the *British Medical Journal* for that year, it noted it had itself become 'less active' because of the 'inaction of the opponents of research'. There had been little 'controversy in the newspapers, and all through the country the great advances made in protective medicine due to research were being appreciated and better understood'. The RDS Committee 'hoped that in the coming years there will hardly be any need for disputes with antivivisection societies, and that the society's best opportunities for usefulness will be found in wide, non-aggressive educational work'.[72]

The war was doubtless partly responsible for the cessation of hostilities. Antivivisection risked an unpatriotic flavour, in the light of the suffering multitudes on the battlefield. But considering the general course of events in the years prior to the war – the founding of the RDS, the Tuberculosis Commission, the National Insurance Act, the founding of the MRC, the negotiation of a second Royal Commission – it seems reasonable to conclude that the strategic defence of experimental medicine had achieved a profound victory already by 1913. The establishment, both medical and lay, political and press, had secured public opinion and the principal of experimental practice against antivivisectionist attacks. The RDS's professions of humanity hit with the

---

[70] Paget to Hale White, 9 October 1916, with RDS Minute of 17 October 1916, Committee minutes from inauguration of RDS, SA/RDS/C/1: Box 2, Wellcome Library London.

[71] Paget to unknown recipient, 21 May 1917, with RDS Minute of 14 May 1917, Committee minutes from inauguration of RDS, SA/RDS/C/1: Box 2, Wellcome Library London.

[72] 'The Research Defence Society', *BMJ*, 14 July 1917.

weight of tacit public approval. A new community of lay actors put their money and their mouths on the line to read the humanitarian script. Medical experimentation as a humane profession was government business, funded by the public purse in the name of the health and fitness of the population at large. It was a new political reality that, paradoxically, allowed the practice of experimentation to operate behind closed doors.

5 Cannon Fire

Drawing Blood

A prone rabbit, bolted to an operating table, stares sightlessly upwards into the glare of an electric light. Above its head a scalpel, held like a pen in the hand of a white-coated, white-bearded physiologist, is poised to make an incision (Figure 5.1).

The raking light illuminates the wraiths of the sick, the physically disabled and the diseased. They are drawn to the scene in the hope of an end to their suffering. These abundant phantoms stalk the physiologist's laboratory: a child on crutches, an ailing baby writhing in the arms of a frantic mother, a blind man. The other faces are those of the poor, whose own lives and the lives of their families are exposed to the ravages of polio, diphtheria, tuberculosis and a host of other diseases. They yearn for security, for vaccines, sera, and curative medicines, and their hopes lie at the sharp edge of the scientist's scalpel. They plead, this band of 'Sufferers': 'For Humanity's Sake, Go On!'

Across the other side of the operating table, in the dark shadows that stand for ignorance, the well-to-do make their protestations in small numbers. The ladies, who are in the majority, are bedecked in fur tippets and muffs, and adorned with the plumes of rare birds. The lone gentleman of the elite stands effetely to the rear, motioning in kid gloves. This group of 'Sentimentalists', who literally wear their general lack of concern for animals, demand hysterically of the physiologist: 'For Mercy's Sake, Stop!'

Central to the piece the physiologist is distracted, annoyed, delayed in his work. His assistant too finds the clamour over his shoulder difficult to ignore. The experimental animal, the rabbit on the table, fixed into a holding apparatus, anaesthetized against pain by the assistant, lies motionless and objectified. Nobody's gaze fixates on this instrumental being. Indeed, it is the only emotionless entity in the room. It feels nothing at the centre of the hubbub.

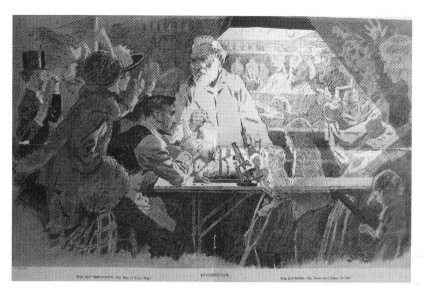

Figure 5.1 'Vivisection', *Puck*, 1911.

Frederick Schiller Lee, Columbia University's leading physiologist, could barely contain his excitement. The image, which appeared in *Puck* magazine in February 1911, was a corrective, re-orientating the propaganda imagery of antivivisectionism, taking attention away from the plight of the experimental animal, putting the plight of human suffering squarely in the balance against the effeminate sentimentalism of the well-to-do. Reframed in this way, antivivisection itself seemed cruel and misguided. Its cries for mercy seemed misplaced, and its campaigners did not seem to understand mercy at all. The day after it appeared, Lee wrote a note to Simon Flexner, Director of the Rockefeller Institute for Medical Research in New York, to tell him about the 'ripping cartoon and editorial on our side', and suggested that they 'get a lot of copies'.[1]

Puck was a major weekly humour and satire outfit, and one of its principal artists, Will Crawford (1869–1944), had apparently reached a perfect understanding of the position carved out by medical scientists over the previous few years, independent of any interference from the medical community. The propaganda value of his artwork was immeasurable. On receipt of Lee's note, Flexner jotted instructions on it and passed it on to Jerome

[1] Lee to Flexner, 23 February 1911, Box 2, FA808, Series 2, Business Manager Correspondence, Rockefeller University Records (RUR), Rockefeller Archive Center, New York (RAC).

Greene (1874–1959), the business manager (from 1910) of the Rockefeller, to do what Lee had asked. 'On behalf of all who believe in the humanity of purpose which dominates research in this country ... I beg to thank you for the affective help you have given',[2] Greene wrote to the publishers of *Puck*. Greene immediately ordered 100 copies of the issue, cash on delivery, and asked for a quote to reprint the page in question 5000 or 10 000 times.[3]

Crawford, the artist, was not finished. A second image, with which this book began (Figure 0.1), cast the ravages of disease among the densely populated quarters of the Lower East Side of Manhattan as a raging conflagration. And in a third image, Figure 5.2, the Sick battles Death in the gladiatorial amphitheatre, and it is from the *hoi polloi* that Death takes his cue. There is nothing automatic about the coup de grace here, disarmed and emasculated as the Sick is. His final appeal to the crowd, again comprising society women with lapdogs, cats, rabbits and rodents – indications of indulgent pity and sentimentalism – falls on deaf ears. The laureled patrician signals thumbs down in accord with the popular clamour. All this takes place in the name of antivivisection, the banner of which is unfurled from the arena wall. Its central symbol is the oil-lamp of progress, burning brightly, but about to be snuffed out by the refined hand of society, pinkie finger extended as a show of urbane form rather than moral substance.

Seen as a triptych, these images hinge on a common perception that the meaning of, and feelings and practices associated with mercy were up for grabs. In each case, the medical practice at the heart of experimental research, principally *cutting*, but encompassing animal experiment in general, whether represented literally, or in the form of a life net, or as sanctioned by political authority, is put forward as authentic mercy, as true humanity, against the feminine cries of those whose attachment to an aesthetics of mercy actually invites suffering and death. The mercy for which the images make an intellectual and practical case is a far-seeing one, pointed at the distant object of public health. The campaign to convince the public that medical research using live animals was *good*, a supreme labour in the name of mercy, hinged on the extent to which such practices could be finessed so as to appear as practices of a particularly masculine medical humanity.

This chapter casts back from this moment in 1911 to the formation of a formal strategic defence of medical research in the USA, making good on the ad hoc, reactionary work and individualized preparation carried out by men like Bowditch and Ernst. It incorporates the opening of the Rockefeller

[2] Greene to Keppler and Schwarzmann, 24 February 1911, Folder 13, Box 5, FA142, Antivivisection Activities, RUR, RAC.
[3] Greene received a quote for $150 for 5,000 copies and $250 for 10,000 copies. It is not clear if he ordered them, though it seems likely.

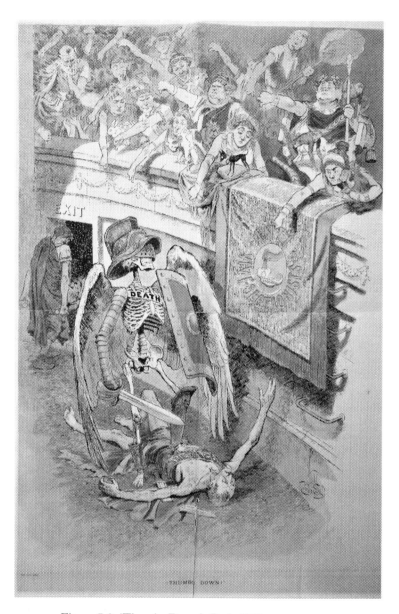

Figure 5.2 'Thumbs Down', *Puck*, 1911.

Institute, the establishment of the Council for the Defense of Medical Research of the American Medical Association, and the development of an art – sometimes literally – of public relations by the medical establishment to protect its scientific methods. In some ways, the *Puck* images represent a major sign of success for the medical scientists' campaign, yet by no means did it signal the end of the struggle. The chapter therefore also casts forward, to the ongoing battles and the further entrenchment of the figure of medical humanity, which would gain new import after the outbreak of war in 1914.

Council for the Defense: Opening Salvos

The Rockefeller Institute was founded in 1901, backed by John D. Rockefeller Sr's (1839–1937) philanthropic notion that medical science could prevent and/or cure diseases that otherwise ravaged the population. Simon Flexner, one of William H. Welch's 'rabbits' at Baltimore, was appointed its Director, and Flexner assembled a team of able experimental professionals. Many of that team would go on to achieve international renown. After years spent buying up equipment, a library, and making ready the Institute's premises on Avenue A (York Avenue) and Sixty-Sixth Street in New York City, the laboratories finally opened in 1906.[4]

This kind of institution existed elsewhere. Europe, as we have seen, was at . the forefront of specialized, professional experimental research involving animals and the concomitant development of research laboratories.[5] The Pasteur Institute in Paris was founded in 1888, and Robert Koch had founded the Royal Prussian Institute for Infectious Diseases (now the Koch Institute) in 1891 in Berlin. At the same time, in London, the British Institute of Preventive Medicine had been opened (subsequently to become the Jenner and latterly the Lister Institute).[6] The Americans were certainly behind in this respect, but the opening of the Rockefeller marked a profound catching up. Within a few years, it would be the pre-eminent

---

[4] Histories of the Rockefeller have tended towards the 'official' in tenor, but they remain invaluable introductions. See George W. Corner, *A History of the Rockefeller Institute 1901–1953, Origins and Growth* (New York: Rockefeller Institute Press, 1964); *Institute to University: A Seventy-Fifth Anniversary Colloquium, June 8, 1976* (New York: Rockefeller University, 1976); Darwin H. Stapleton, ed., *Creating a Tradition of Biomedical Research: Contributions to the History of the Rockefeller University* (New York: Rockefeller University Press, 2004).

[5] Andrew Cunningham and Perry Williams, eds, *The Laboratory Revolution in Medicine* (Cambridge: Cambridge University Press, 1992).

[6] The British Institute's new premises in Chelsea had been protested by local residents in 1894, who worried about howling 'all night long', bad smells, and the 'cruel shame' of experimenting on dogs. Wellcome Library, London, Lister Institute Collection, Vivisection Controversy Section, SA/LIS/E.3, 'Report of survey of residents in Chelsea Gardens re proposed Institute'.

medical research facility in the world, not least because it was so well funded. A research hospital was attached to the Institute by 1910, and a separate animal facility was opened in Princeton in 1914. Its staff became experts at staving off legislation that would hurt them, drawing up new legislation that would help them, influencing public opinion in innovative ways that marked a sea-change in medical public-relations machinery and its application, and all the while conducted experimental research that would, in its early years, have a dramatic impact on public health in America and beyond.

Yet insofar as the Rockefeller shifted the vanguard of medical research to New York, it also moved with it the cause of international antivivisection. New York was to be the front line for arguments for and against animal experimentation. After the Rockefeller opened in 1906 there was a flurry of activity. In 1907, in Brooklyn, the Society for the Prevention of Abuse in Animal Experimentation was formed. The following year saw the foundation of the New York Anti-Vivisection Society. Also in 1908, the American Society for the Prevention of Cruelty to Animals, which had long been silent on the question of vivisection, deferring to the status and expertise of medical men, supported a Bill to regulate vivisection activity that went before the New York State Legislature. Such Bills would be relaunched in 1909, 1910, 1911 and 1912. It has been pointed out by historians of antivivisection that much of this activity was not staunchly abolitionist, but reformist.[7] Following the English model, which had subjected animal experimentation to a State-managed licensing system since 1876, the major goal of the antivivisection movement was to establish external regulation and oversight of medical activity.

These moderate aims notwithstanding, the medical establishment saw such attempts as the thin end of the wedge. Whatever the apparent moderation in the Legislature, the public discourse fuelling such efforts, especially in the pages of *The New York Herald*, which had taken the side of the New York Anti-Vivisection Society and offered a platform to its chief agitator, Diana Belais (1858–1944), was nothing if not radical. The noise easily drowned out the nuanced middle ground. The loudest voices were those of prominent female activists, such as Lizzie Lind af Hageby and Caroline Earl White, along with Belais. The medical establishment understood those voices to be an hysterical expression of aesthetic sentimentalism (irrespective of how those women saw themselves and the nature of their campaign). It became a major focus of the medical response to meet those voices with an opposing sober masculinity,

---

[7] Bernard Unti, "'The Doctors Are So Sure That They Only Are Right': The Rockefeller Institute and the Defeat of Vivisection Reform in New York, 1908–1914', in Stapleton, *Creating a Tradition*, 175–8.

building upon the, by then, well-founded scientific sense of 'humanity' without reference to sentiment.[8]

In April 1908, Stephen Paget wrote to Walter Cannon at Harvard, expressing a hope that a 'sister Society' to his own Research Defence Society would 'be founded in America'.[9] By that time, Paget had already been in touch with Simon Flexner, Harvey Cushing and others. When, in May 1908, William H. Welch wrote to Simon Flexner and confessed to 'thinking that probably the time has come to establish a research defence society', the idea was already maturing among the medical establishment. Welch was not necessarily convinced. Until that time, the efforts of individuals and the loose network of medical scientists had sufficed to keep antivivisection at bay, focusing on preventing legislation by direct remonstrance.[10] Welch thought that corporate opinion on 'agitation of the subject in the public press' was undesirable because it recognized the 'strength of the opposition'. Welch was altogether sanguine about the 'minds of the intelligent public', who could decide for themselves that what they saw in organs such as the *New York Herald* was nothing less than 'villainous'. Always in the minds of the American medical community was the British Act of 1876, against which and through which they had to practice, and Welch at least thought that a defence society might prompt the lay community, on whose public opinion the freedom of medical research relied, to initiate proactive attempts to legislate medical research from within. For Welch and others, such a prospect of any inroads into the liberty of research was abhorrent. Welch thought that without a 'large body of influential and eminent laymen, it would not be worth while . . . to establish the society'.[11] He had in mind prominent clergymen, university presidents, judges and so on. Something similar to this notion was also in the mind of George Simmons, General Secretary of the American Medical Association, and himself a major force behind the popularization of medical science in the early twentieth century. Under his editorship, the *Journal of the American Medical Association* soared from about 1000 to about 80 000 subscribers, and it would become the venue for much of the

---

[8] It was even pathologized. See Craig Buettinger, 'Antivivisection and the Charge of Zoophil-Psychosis in the Early Twentieth Century', *The Historian*, 55 (1992): 277–88. Buettinger opines that 'When challenged by the lay and predominantly female antivivisection movement, scientists brimmed with condescension and misogyny; and, in the case of the zoophil-psychosis concept, so too did their science', and I take his point. But it is also important not to reduce the defence of vivisection in this period to misogyny.

[9] Paget to Cannon, April 1908, H MS c 40, Folder 340, Box 28, WBCA. For Paget's English Research Defence Society, see Chapter 4.

[10] The subject of Chapter 3.

[11] Welch to Flexner, 19 May 1908, Reel 7, FA746, Series 1, Simon Flexner Papers; Subseries 1.1 Personal Papers, Simon Flexner Papers (American Philosophical Society), RAC.

Council for Defense's literature in praise of animal experimentation. Simmons felt any medical propaganda campaign would be 'much more effective if laymen were on the Council'.[12]

It seems Welch's younger colleagues did not share these views, or see a future for American medical research along anything like the same lines as the British case. Cannon had first entered the fray in 1906, to combat Senate Bill 99 in Massachusetts. At that stage, Harold Ernst's coordination of the defence came with a great sense of personal imposition, and it was clear that a new general was going to be necessary in forthcoming battles (see Chapter 3). Cannon – a mentee of Bowditch and the successor to his physiological laboratory at Harvard – fired his first volley then, which was to be the first shot in a generation-long barrage. Cannon wrote Paget on 20 May 1908 to intimate that the Americans were about to undertake 'a campaign of education' and to say that the time had come 'for this movement in the United States'. To Paget he expressed a hope that the two societies could mutually benefit each other, but the vision for the American society was starkly different to that of Paget's.[13] Cannon relayed Paget's formulation that 'a doctor counts one, a layman counts two, a lady counts three, and a cleric counts four', to Lee at Columbia, but pointed out that American conditions, at least from his perspective, were different. The medical profession in America had a greater reputation, and America benefitted from having no established church to meddle in 'legislative affairs'.[14] Cannon told Simmons that he had sounded his colleagues on the matter and decided that 'it seems desirable to work through the medical profession'.[15] It was a position that the Council stuck to over years, despite repeated calls from significant medical figures such as William Williams Keen, and it transpired to be justified in the continued success of the medical profession in defeating antivivisectionist moves against them.[16]

---

[12] Simmons to Cannon, 26 August 1908, H MS c 40, Folder 333, Box 28, WBCA.

[13] Cannon to Paget, 20 May 1908, H MS c 40, Folder 340, Box 28, WBCA.

[14] Cannon to Lee, 8 December 1908, H MS c 40, Folder 339, Box 28, WBCA. It is remarkable that the Americans took little if any note of the British Association for the Advancement of Medicine by Research, or the extent to which the medical establishment had, through this body, effectively controlled the administration of the law that was rhetorically so often maligned. While 1876 was presented by Paget et al. as a disaster, it had been Paget, and his father before him, who had in fact ensured that the Act was no great barrier to experimental research through the AAMR.

[15] Cannon to Simmons, 24 August 1908, H MS c 40, Folder 333, Box 28, WBCA.

[16] William H. Welch set out all of the principal arguments against a lay society after the English fashion in a letter to Flexner in 1908. Welch to Flexner, 27 May 1908, Reel 7, FA746, Series 1 Simon Flexner Papers; Subseries 1.1 Personal Papers, Simon Flexner Papers (American Philosophical Society), RAC. In the case of Keen, the topic of a lay society, to be formulated on a national basis, was raised in 1913, and Keen summoned all the principal men to Philadelphia to discuss the issue. It is clear from correspondence that

A flurry of activity in the middle of 1908 brought the Council for the Defense of Medical Research (CDMR) of the American Medical Association into being.[17] Cannon, as probably the nation's leading physiologist, and as the heir to the oldest struggles with antivivisection in America, was brought to the fore by Welch and Simmons and recruited to lead the Council's activities. Other members of the council included J. A. Capps of Chicago, Harvey Cushing of Baltimore, David Edsall (1869–1945) of Philadelphia, Simon Flexner of New York, Reid Hunt (1870–1948) of Washington and Herbert Moffitt (1867–1950) of San Francisco. In short, the Council comprised a who's who of American physiology and animal experimentation. Cannon's primary task, which he set about with great energy, was to establish contact with medical schools across the country, asking them by circular letter about their experiences with animal experimentation. This was to be reinforced by personal visits from Dr N. P. Colwell, Secretary of the Council on Medical Education of the AMA, who was to visit the nation's schools over a period of years. The Council was satisfied by the responses it received from around the country that there was a high standard of ethical practice already in place, and that laboratories were perfectly capable of self-regulation.[18] As early as

there was little appeal. Flexner at the Rockefeller certainly demurred, and the Institute's business manager, Henry James Jr, agreed that 'this idea of Keen's is a mistake', principally because the presence of a national society would make 'everything put out in defense of research' look like an 'organized effort', and dismissed as partisan. The subtle, back-channel working of editorial relationships was far more sophisticated, but it seems that Keen had no real appreciation of the front-line work being undertaken in New York and Boston. See James Jr to Flexner (no date), appended to Keen to Flexner, 10 December 1913, Reel 59, FA746, Series 1, Simon Flexner Papers; Subseries 1.2, Rockefeller Institute for Medical Research, Simon Flexner Papers (American Philosophical Society), RAC. When a lay society was eventually formed, in 1923, it realized many of Flexner's fears. See Karen D. Ross, 'Recruiting "Friends of Medical Progress": Evolving Tactics in the Defense of Animal Experimentation, 1910s and 1920s', *Journal of the History of Medicine and Allied Sciences*, 70 (2015): 365–93.

[17] For general coverage of this period, see Susan Lederer, 'The Controversy over Animal Experimentation in America, 1880–1914', in *Vivisection in Historical Perspective*, ed. Nicolaas Rupke (London: Croom Helm, 1987). The CDMR itself is surprisingly under researched. The primary body of sources relating to its foundation and strategic operation is held at the Countway Library of Medicine in Boston, among the Cannon papers. The go-to secondary source would be Susan Lederer's landmark *Subjected to Science: Human Experimentation in America before the Second World War* (Baltimore: Johns Hopkins University Press, 1995), which begins much where this book ends. Lederer only references the Cannon papers a handful of times in that book. Other works, much more specifically about the CDMR and this small flashpoint of history concerning medical research, make no reference to the Cannon papers whatsoever: Mary L. Westermann-Cicio, 'Of Mice and Medical Men: The Medical Profession's Response to the Vivisection Controversy in Turn of the Century America', PhD thesis, State University of New York (2001).

[18] Welch to Cannon, 3 July 1908; Simmons to Cannon, 10 July 1908; Cannon to Colwell, 23 November 1908; Colwell to Cannon, 25 November 1908; Cannon to Colwell, 27 November 1908, H MS c 40, Folder 332, Box 28, WBCA.

February 1909, Cannon could write to Paget in England to reassure him of the 'thoroughly justifiable attitude toward animal experimentation' that prevailed in medical schools all through the USA. Students were informed of the 'importance of the experimental method' and they were warned 'not to do anything that would in any way tend to arouse public opinion against it'. Most laboratories already boasted their own rules of procedure, a departure of some significance since the time Ernst had asked the same question, with a strict emphasis on humane ethics. To make sure there could be little complaint, the Council drew up a list of rules to be posted in laboratories, ensuring a certain minimum standard of practice when employing experimental animals for research. These were collated, revised, and distributed by the CDMR so that all medical schools and laboratories were following the same principles of practice.[19] For Cannon and the other Council members, there is no sense that this was a cynical strategy of managing the optics of animal experimentation. They considered themselves exceptionally humane men, hurt all the more by accusations of inhumanity.[20]

Nonetheless, a certain air of calculation was essential to the Council's success. Coordinating with the Committee of Medical Legislation of the AMA, it was to be informed of any proposed antivivisection legislation anywhere in the country, so that it could act accordingly in good time.[21] This was reinforced by an informal correspondence network, with major nodes of communication resting with Cannon in Boston and with Flexner (and his business managers, Jerome Greene and then Henry James Jr) at the Rockefeller Institute in New York. Everywhere that there was antivivisection activity, there were medical informants or their agents in attendance. The channels of intelligence sharing were open, slick and effective.

In addition – and this had been Cannon's main initiative in seeing the purpose of a Council in the first place – a series of articles were to be written in defence of animal experimentation, to be published in esteemed journals, the content of which could then be boiled down and relayed to the popular press. Through the instruments of the AMA, Cannon could get a press release out to some 5000 newspapers or other media in quick time. In all of

---

[19] Cannon to Colwell, 21 January 1909, H MS c 40, Folder 332, Box 28; Cannon to Paget, 18 February 1909, H MS c 40, Folder 340, Box 28, WBCA. For the rules, see Walter B. Cannon, 'Medical Control of Vivisection', *North American Review*, 191 (1910): 817.

[20] Cannon's overall liberal humanitarian credentials would become a noted part of his career. He would go on to become chairman of the American Medical Bureau to Aid Spanish Democracy. See Aelwen D. Wetherby, *Private Aid, Political Activism: American Medical Relief to Spain and China, 1936–1949* (Columbia: University of Missouri Press, 2017).

[21] Frederick R. Green to Cannon, 30 November 1908 and 7 December 1908; George W. Gay to Cannon, 14 December 1908, H MS c 40, Folder 332, Box 28, WBCA.

this communication, the Council resolved to avoid sensationalism on its part and to side-step what it saw as the sentimentalism of the other side. Education was to be sober, though by no means were the Council's activities lacking in affective pleading.[22] In these matters, the Board of Public Instruction of the AMA deferred entirely to the new Council.

At the core of the new Council's activities, therefore, was the wielding of the power and influence that inhered in medical credibility. It was to be applied in two directions: towards thwarting the legislative attempts of antivivisection, and towards influencing public opinion without appearing directly to be manipulating the press in a conscious campaign. Both of these strategies would turn out to be highly successful. The fact that the medical establishment was able to secure much of the mainstream press in its favour, without the need for prominent members of the lay public to intercede, was a major achievement unmatched in Britain.

Yet for all the new Council set out to co-ordinate a defence strategy across the USA, its principal focus was always New York. Even when flashpoints of controversy occurred elsewhere – in Philadelphia, or in Washington, DC – it was the New York scientists, at the Rockefeller and at Columbia, who were the chief informants, organizers and, in the press, the public voices of the humanity of medical research. Insofar as Cannon in Boston was often the one to fire volleys on behalf of the medical community and beyond, it was just as often that Flexner, Lee, et al, supplied the ammunition.

The necessity of CDMR's work quickly became self-evident, and its capacity to draw upon international experience and networks of intelligence became invaluable. In January 1909, Paget wrote to Cannon, having read that Lind af Hageby had sailed on the *Mauretania* for New York, with the intent of carrying on her antivivisection campaign there. Paget supplied Cannon with chapter and verse on her activities, propaganda, first libel trial, relationship with Stephen Coleridge (who would also execute an American antivivisection lecture tour) and her general approach.[23] But such was the state of vigilance among the medical research community, Paget's letter found Cannon not only already prepared, but already engaged in a quiet manipulation of public opinion on the matter. Flexner had written in early December 1908, telling Cannon that 'we should start in at once to circulate through the press information concerning' Coleridge and Lind af Hageby's careers. He added, 'the active elements among the physicians should be organized against the movement ... they could bring pressure to

[22] Cannon to John G. Clark, 16 November 1908, 14 December 1908; Clark to Cannon, 12 December 1908, H MS c 40, Folder 332, Box 28, WBCA.
[23] Paget to Cannon, 30 January 1909, H MS c 40, Folder 340, Box 28, WBCA.

bear on a good class of citizens as well as on the legislator'.[24] Before Lind af Hageby's arrival, therefore, Cannon had already circulated 'a brief account of her career' to Lee in New York and Edsall in Philadelphia, which was subsequently forwarded to the press so 'that the papers knew her untrustworthiness'.[25]

The results were a clear victory for black operations. Accounts of Lind af Hageby's addresses in New York, at the Carnegie Lyceum, sponsored by the New York Anti-Vivisection Society, were reported in the *New York Times* and the *Sun*, immediately followed by critical commentary by Lee. The *New York Times* ran the story under the headline, 'Heckled Miss Lind, Anti-Vivisectionist', and noted one of her characteristic arguments that sentimentalism was no ground for dismissal of her views, since 'all the world was sentiment, and that many of the best things of the world ... were founded on sentiment'. This did not prevent her from repeating the libel against W. M. Bayliss and the whole 'Brown Dog Affair', and nor did it prevent her making the extraordinary claim that vivisection 'created a taste' for such experiments among students, 'till frequently human beings, who were poor and helpless, were experimented upon in similar manner'.[26] Lee's commentary almost served to concede Lind's point about sentiment. He did not question her 'sincerity', but rather the 'quality and trustworthiness' of her leadership of the movement. After all, Lind was a proven liar, anti-science *tout court*, and was easily condemned out of her own mouth.[27] *Collier's Weekly* – a known ally of medical science – treated the addresses, and Lind's appearances, as so much editorial meat to chew, repeating much that had been circulated by Cannon, including the contrite statement of Lind's publisher, when forced to withdraw Lind's libellous *Shambles of Science*. Repeating Lind's statements could be dangerous, *Collier's* warned: 'Save your money: you may need it' to pay damages for libel![28] In Philadelphia, the *North American* initially perturbed the scientists, running an interview with Lind and a prominent account of her address there. Cannon reported that 'Dr. Edsall felt that his efforts had been in vain',

[24] Flexner to Cannon, 9 December 1908, H MS c 40, Folder 336, Box 28, WBCA.

[25] Cannon to Paget, 18 February 1909, H MS c 40, Folder 340, Box 28, WBCA. Cannon's letter to Lee, with a full brief on Lind af Hageby's life and career, is dated 21 January 1909, H MS c 40, Folder 339, Box 28, WBCA. Lee's intention to brief the dailies is stated in Lee to Cannon, 29 January 1909, H MS c 40, Folder 339, Box 28, WBCA. Edsall's arrangements with the press in Philadelphia are stated in Cannon to Lee, 30 January 1909, H MS c 40, Folder 339, Box 28, WBCA.

[26] *New York Times*, 4 February 1909. (Lind af Hageby's English activities are the subject of part of Chapter 4.)

[27] F. S. Lee to the Editor of the *New York Times*, *New York Times*, 4 February 1909.

[28] 'The Lady and the Truth', *Collier's*, 13 February 1909, 10. It was clear that Lee knew in advance that *Collier's* would run the story: Lee to Cannon, 29 January 1909, H MS c 49, Folder 339, Box 28, WBCA.

but it transpired that the paper was 'merely arousing interest. The next day a very affecting letter from a father whose children were miraculously saved from diphtheria was published with prominent headlines, and on Monday a long editorial (the only editorial) was printed countering squarely on Miss Lind and her contentions'.[29] These opening salvos were to become representative of the CDMR's general strategy of meeting the challenges of its opponents in public. Direct engagement was deferred in favour of indirect influence of the press, which, through such profoundly popular organs as the *New York Times* and *Collier's*, was great indeed.

In private correspondence, true feelings about these activists were aired, in a manner far removed from the way they were publicly addressed. Coleridge, for example, was 'a slippery unscrupulous person', according to Cannon. Tongue in cheek, Cannon referred to the cruelty of Lind's barbs, musing that it 'might be well to urge her stewards take care to anaesthetize her opponents before doing them injury'.[30] The community of medical scientists in America, by and large, thought their opponents were cranks and hypocrites, ignorant, sentimental, vainglorious attention seekers. The trick was to persuade the public of this without resorting to name-calling.

Heart Work

In 1909, William Williams Keen documented for the popular press a new chapter in 'the happy history of progress'. It was a heart-stopping moment, literally. Three years previously, he had witnessed George Washington Crile 'chloroform a dog to death' with the express purpose of reanimating it. The moment its heart ceased to beat was recorded accurately and then Keen checked his watch, telling off fifteen minutes before Crile injected the dog's heart with saline and adrenalin. A few chest compressions later and the dog was 'as much alive as he had been a half-hour before'. Thereby, the 'immense value' of the adrenal gland was revealed.[31]

As the defence of experimental medicine in the USA became more organized, it continued to take place on three fronts: laboratory practices, legislative remonstrances and public representation. In each case, the work undertaken was another kind of heart work: an exercise in 'emotional labour' to bring about a set of desired feelings in association with a set of predefined activities.[32] Here I borrow a phrase from Arlie Russel

---

[29] Cannon to Paget, 18 February 1909, H MS c 40, Folder 340, Box 28, WBCA.

[30] Cannon to Paget, 18 February 1909, H MS c 40, Folder 340, Box 28, WBCA.

[31] W. W. Keen, 'Recent Surgical Progress: A Result Chiefly of Experimental Research', *Harper's Monthly*, 118 (1909): 765.

[32] Arlie Russel Hochschild, *The Managed Heart: Commercialization of Human Feeling* (Berkeley: University of California Press, 1983).

Hochschild and extend its meaning. In its original usage, Hochschild referred to the ways in which prescribed expressions served to inculcate the emotion displayed, such that inducements to smile resulted in happy feelings, for example.[33] The three fronts here – of experiment, legal defence and representation – amount to emotive practices to forge a desired feeling. The practice of medical research was an exercise in the direct experience of medical compassion at a stage of remove from its implementation in the world. Keen's account of Crile's adrenalin experiments are a case in point. The experiment necessitated killing a dog, but Keen was careful to point out two things: the dog was under anaesthetic (indeed, was killed by it), and reanimated without it yet becoming conscious. It therefore did not suffer. And the experiment revealed an immeasurably useful medical application for humans and animals alike. This was practical beneficence. It was a 'happy' story. Practice connected an intellectual conviction (that medical research was humanitarian in its intent) with knowledge of the successful application of previous research (proof of the concept of humanitarianism). It was fundamentally about exercising the principle that experimentation, including cutting and killing, was a moral good. Defending medical research against legal inroads was about projecting the humanitarian benefits of research onto legislators, while preserving knowledge of this specialist practice of that humanitarianism as inaccessible to anybody but experts. It sought to demonstrate that appeals for reform of the animal cruelty laws came from a place of misunderstanding and emotional inadequacy (sentimentalism), while asking legislators to take *on trust* the humanitarian feeling of medical researchers. This trust was principally acquired obliquely, by reference to the proven human benefits of scientific work. Nonetheless, for all that medical scientists remonstrated on grounds of legal technicality, their emotional labour here was intentional: it sought to inculcate trust in medical scientists among non-medical professionals. The representative, media work also aimed at building trust in the lay public, utilizing the social

---

[33] This sociological study has since been re-imagined by psychologists and labelled the 'facial feedback hypothesis', namely that the experience of emotion is coloured by 'feedback' from facial movement. See, for example, Nicholas A. Coles, Jeff T. Larsen and Heather C. Lench, 'A Meta-Analysis of the Facial Feedback Literature: Effects of Facial Feedback on Emotional Experience Are Small and Variable', *Psychological Bulletin* (2019). Here I take a somewhat broader view, which is to imagine scientists not merely expressing the emotions they desired to experience, either facially or bodily or even verbally, but, as per Hochschild's study, expressing these emotions in a collective context of mutual reinforcement and recapitulation. Scientific practice, in this case, is indistinguishable from its associated affective practices of expressing/emoting, in order to give a consistency of meaning to the experience of scientific practice. Such practice therefore becomes a mode of *doing* emotion, such that rehearsals of the expression of the desired emotion – here mercy, sympathy, humanity – end up feeding back upon the lived experience of the practice so that experimentation becomes lived humanitarianism.

status and professional respect accorded to MDs, as had been done with the legislators, but going further, towards the making of medical heroes. The second and third of these fronts were, in their attempts to alter the emotions of others and to influence the reception of medical science, dynamically reflexive. Through the success that the medical establishment had in both of these areas, it was further confirmed in the moral virtue of medical research as a humanitarian practice, experienced first-hand only in the laboratory.

The core strategy of the CDMR concerned public education, and insofar as there was a strategic plan it involved coordinated efforts in the realm of representation. But the specific need for particular types of representation arose in the light of new legislative challenges and as new techniques and medical applications were developed in practice. More importantly, the sense of an acute need for positive representation – for dynamic emotional labour in the press – arose in the face of denunciation and defamation from antivivisectionists, which threatened the reputation and purpose of medical research unpredictably. As such, I have attempted here to put forward the experience of medical research as a complex and messy whole. What follows, therefore, is an appraisal of the affective character of the defence of research, and implicitly, an account of the lived experience of that defence.

At an individual level, medical scientists experienced this as a sort of quotidian satisfaction, as an important job, done well.[34] The experimental success of the Rockefeller staff, for example, of Flexner himself who created a protective serum against meningitis, of men like Hideyo Noguchi (1876–1928) who thought he had contrived a new way to test for syphilis, and of Alexis Carrel (1873–1944), whose refined surgical techniques were won at the expense of many a laboratory animal, was – in their own minds – the product of simple procedure and honest toil.[35] The

---

[34] For the emotional management of animal experimentation (both the experimenter's emotions and the animal's), and its contrast with the emotional investments of antivivisectionists, see Otniel Dror, 'The Affect of Experiment: The Turn to Emotions in Anglo-American Physiology, 1900–1940', *Isis*, 90 (1999): 236.

[35] The controversy surrounding Noguchi's syphilis work, which generated a recurring cycle of accusations of human experimentation, especially on children, has been extensively analysed. See Susan Lederer, 'Hideyo Noguchi's Luetin Experiment and the Antivivisectionists', *Isis*, 76 (1985): 31–48. For a more general appraisal of his career, see Aya Takahashi, 'Hideyo Noguchi, the Pursuit of Immunity and the Persistence of Fame: A Reappraisal', in Stapleton, *Creating a Tradition*, 227–39. For Carrel, see Shelley McKellar, 'Innovation in Modern Surgery: Alexis Carrel and Blood Vessel Repair', in Stapleton, *Creating a Tradition*, 135–50; David M. Friedman, *The Immortalists; Charles Lindbergh, Dr. Alexis Carrel, and Their Daring Quest to Live Forever* (New York: Harper, 2007); Hannah Landecker, *Culturing Life: How Cells Became Technologies* (Cambridge, MA: Harvard University Press, 2007), 68–92. For Flexner, see Saul Benison, 'Simon Flexner: The Evolution of a Career in Medical Science', in *Institute to University*, 13–35;

exchange of correspondence in the light of Carrel being awarded the Nobel Prize in 1912, for example, is telling. The notice from the Carolin Institute that awarded him the prize connected animal experimentation and the development of surgery as an applied science, congratulating Carrel on pursuing his 'distinct end ... without respite'.[36] Cannon congratulated him on his recognition 'after years of detraction and incredulity and from some quarters ridicule', but told him not to reply to his letter because 'you have more important work to do. With best wishes for the continued success of that work'.[37] Carrel himself refused most of the offers he received to flaunt his work after the award of the prize, on the basis that he had too much work to do.[38]

Flexner summed up the atmosphere of research as follows: 'it is our purpose, through medical research, to protect human life', and he happened 'to be one of those men' whose whole life was dedicated to that object. 'I have', he said, 'spent all my prifessional [sic] life at that job'.[39] Others clearly comprehended the entanglement of scientific effort and humanitarian ends. One correspondent to the New York Times demanded that New Yorkers 'help to preserve the conditions under which alone he [Flexner] can hope to pursue his labors. They can protect him against interruption and annoyance; against the necessity of devoting part of his precious time and energy to combating efforts to tie his hands. Every moment taken from his work is to that extent a limitation upon scientific effort in behalf of humanity'.[40]

Together the Rockefeller staff call to mind the speech of English scientist and public-health pioneer John Simon at the IMC in 1881, when he declared that medical scientists' 'verb of life is [to work], not [to feel]'.[41] Laboratory work was a practice of humanity that was experienced simply as work. And of course, the Rockefeller was emblematic of a general trend across the institutions of medical science in the USA. The 1913 resolutions adopted by the Federation of American Societies for Experimental Biology,

for a general account, see James Thomas Flexner, *An American Saga: The Story of Helen Thomas and Simon Flexner* (New York: Fordham University Press, 1993).

[36] Translation, citation accompanying the award of the Nobel Prize to Doctor Carrel, Folder 8, Box 2, Series 2: Carrel Files, Theodore Malinin collection of Alexis Carrel and Charles Lindbergh papers, RAC.

[37] Cannon to Carrel, 3 October 1912, Folder 32, Box 2, FA208, Series 2: Carrel Files, Theodor Malinin collection of Alexis Carrel and Charles Lindbergh papers, RAC.

[38] The tenor of much of his general correspondence for 1912, Series 2: Carrel Files, Theodore Malinin collection of Alexis Carrel and Charles Lindbergh papers, RAC.

[39] Hearing before the Senate Judiciary Committee and Assembly Committee/Public Health, Albany, New York, 8 March 1911, Folder 21, Box 2, FA142, Anti-vivisection Activities, RUR, RAC.

[40] James P. Harrison to the *New York Times*, clipping, Folder 1, Box 16, FA142, Anti-vivisection activities, RUR, RAC.

[41] See Chapter 1.

for example – a federation comprising the American Physiological Society, the American Society for Biological Chemists, the American Society for Pharmacology and Experimental Therapeutics, and the American Society for Experimental Pathology – included the following self-description: medical experimenters were 'self-sacrificing, high-minded men of science who are devoting their lives to the welfare of mankind in efforts to solve the complicated problems of living beings and their diseases'.[42]

That medical scientists, whose work depended on the experimental destruction of animals, could really have been, or believed themselves to be, hard-working humanitarians, should be credited. The power of rhetoric, intertwined with practice, and compounded by the production of evidence, *makes* the experience so described. The humanitarian intent of medical scientists, and therefore their experience of their work as a humanitarian practice, should be taken seriously. Witness, for example, the statement of John W. Churchman (d. 1937), instructor in surgery at Johns Hopkins: 'in communities where experimentation is going on it is to those interested in animal investigation that the profession looks for leadership in its far-sighted campaign for health and happiness of this and future generations'. They were a community 'busy with intelligent philanthropy'.[43] We can argue the merits of that philanthropy, perhaps, but not its lived, situated reality.

Walter Cannon, to take a more prominent example, was also deeply persuaded of the humanity of his own practices and of those of his colleagues. Since the procedural rules of laboratories were to be overseen and upheld by the directors of those laboratories, there could be little doubt as to their being carefully observed. Such men, after all, were men 'of prominence in the profession and in the community'. If anything, in Cannon's eyes, this guarantee of ethical observance was far more satisfactory than any occasional third-party inspector's report could ever be. The 'educational process' that the CDMR was setting in motion was a 'slow one', but Cannon felt it 'fundamental' and was assured that, in the end, it would 'result in registering the common sense of sane people'.[44] Here was the nub of the argument: antivivisectionists could not be classified among the sane, whereas the super sanity of medical science was often lost on the public because of the high degree of specialism in its knowledge creation and procedures. The battle, therefore, was for the hearts and minds of the sane laity. That battle hinged, as Cannon himself wrote, on cultivating

---

[42] Resolutions adopted by The Federation of American Societies for Experimental Biology, Philadelphia, 31 December 1913, Folder 1, Box 1, FA142, Anti-vivisection Activities, RUR, RAC.

[43] John W. Churchman, 'The Value of Animal Experimentation as Illustrated by Recent Advances in the Study of Syphilis' (Chicago: American Medical Association, 1911), 24.

[44] Cannon to Paget, 18 February 1909, H MS c 40, Folder 340, Box 28, WBCA.

respect for the 'high purpose of biologic investigation and its beneficent achievements for human welfare, which together give meaning and sanction to the experimental use of animals'.[45] While in practice, it also meant keeping antivivisection off the statute books, the recourse to the 'meaning and sanction' of animal experimentation based on its beneficence was an ever present central feature of the medical argument.

Modern Medical Miracles

The American defence of research continued to engage with the law, for the most part, only to prevent legislative innovation. The entire case of the medical establishment was that existing State and Federal laws were already sufficient to police abuse in animal research. Cruelty was cruelty, went the argument, and no further clarification was required to make laboratory cruelty illegal or the path towards correcting injustice open. The whole point was that, by the standards of cruelty spelled out in such legislation, medical researchers were categorically not cruel.[46] Either the animals in their charge were dealt with humanely and painlessly, for the sake of a greater good, or else they were caused pain and suffering with all due sensibility towards such suffering, but with the knowledge of the actual or potential benefits of such actions. As such, medical practice per se could not be considered to be *wanton* in any sense. The factor of deliberation was antithetical to cruelty, as far as medical science was concerned.

In practice this amounted to a continuation of annual battles in State legislatures. The tenor of medical remonstrances against dangerous Bills always emphasized the humanitarian intent of experimenters, as well as recounting the humanitarian benefits already accrued from research. But insofar as they strove to persuade legislators of this, the argument hinged on legal necessity. The best evidence doctors had that experimental medicine was not cruel was the fact that nobody had ever been successfully prosecuted for cruelty in the laboratory, which existing laws would have permitted were there evidence for it. Their argument was that this lack of prosecution was evidence of high-mindedness, not, as the antivivisectors claimed, evidence of the inadequacy of the existing law. By way of

---

[45] Walter B. Cannon, *Some Characteristics of Antivivisection Literature* (Chicago: AMA, 1911), 14.

[46] There was no federal law until 1966, but various state laws existed much earlier, especially in those states – Massachusetts (1835), New York (1828) – that were the main focus of earlier antivivisectionist attention. By 1907, every state in the union had some form of anti-cruelty legislation. See Diane L. Beers, *For the Prevention of Cruelty: The History and Legacy of Animal Rights Activism in the United States* (Ohio: Swallow Press, 2006).

substantiation, therefore, medical remonstrances dwelt at length on medical high-minded humanity and on the quality and efficacy of existing
legislation.[47]

After 1908, however, with the CDMR up and running, the way in which
the medical establishment were strategically mobilized was often more
telling than the specifics of their arguments. As early as March 1909,
Cannon was able to describe to Paget in London the many legislative fronts
upon which the CDMR was fighting – in Pennsylvania, New York,
Wisconsin and so on – and his confidence in the 'machinery' of his organization. Evidence as to the efficacy of existing laws was to be compiled,
printed and distributed throughout the country, so that State Legislatures
could be presented with a ready-made arguments wherever antivivisection
Bills emerged.[48] Medical scientists in different parts of the country tended to
lend this a military air. When Joseph Bryant (1845–1914), prominent
surgeon at New York University, wrote to Simmons at the AMA in
October 1908, his tone was positively belligerent. Concerned at
a prospective Bill against vivisection in the District of Columbia, Bryant
referred to antivivisectionists as 'the enemy' and demanded that the AMA
'get in the field'.[49] Simmons forwarded the letter immediately to Cannon,
who replied detailing the CDMR's strategies of remonstrance and education, with special reference to the 'testimony of prominent men'.[50]

More broadly, however, the medical establishment sough to keep public
opinion on side especially at key moments of legislative debate. After the
end of a season of struggle over the Davis-Lee Bill before the New York
State Legislature in early 1909, for example, Cannon wrote to Lee with
congratulations, noting *en passant* that it was surely no accident that key
supporting articles appeared in important journals, 'timed for the psychological moment in the New York struggle'.[51] The articles in question were
by Burton J. Hendrick (1870–1949) in *McClure's* and by William Williams
Keen in *Harper's Monthly*. In the case of Keen, a prominent medical
scientist himself, the motivation is clear enough. Keen had a rare knack
of being able to write for popular audiences while remaining a lauded
figure in the profession. The title of his piece, 'Recent Surgical Progress:
A Result Chiefly of Experimental Research', could not have more effectively encapsulated the argument. It was subsequently reissued in London,

---

[47] Cannon to Paget, 15 March 1909, H MS c 40, Folder 340, Box 28, WBCA.
[48] Cannon to Paget, 15 March 1909, H MS c 40, Folder 340, Box 28, WBCA.
[49] Bryant to Simmons, 22 October 1908, H MS c 40, Folder 342, Box 28, WBCA.
[50] Cannon to Bryant, 26 October 1908, H MS c 40, Folder 342, Box 28, WBCA.
[51] Cannon to Lee, 26 March 1909, H MS c 40, Folder 339, Box 28, WBCA. The Davis–
Lee Bill had been put forward in 1908, having been written by Frederick Bellamy of the
Society for the Prevention of Abuse in Animal Experimentation. See Unti, 'The Doctors
Are So Sure', 175ff.

under the auspices of Paget's Research Defence Society[52] and published again along with all of Keen's popular writings on the subject in a 1914 volume entitled *Animal Experimentation and Medical Progress*.[53]

We have to dig a little deeper with Hendrick.[54] Hendrick actually wrote two articles for *McClure's Magazine* in 1909. *McClure's Magazine* was a popular monthly, published in New York, known in these years for its investigative journalism. It was editorially disposed in favour of medical science, and Hendrick, one of its chief writers, formed a special attachment to the medical community, especially at the Rockefeller. He was a muckraking journalist, a populist writer, but no man of science. Yet his articles, which defended in close detail the operations of the Rockefeller Institute, were, from the point of view of the medical establishment, perfectly written defences of both the use of animals in experimental research and of the humanity of the men who performed such experiments. The information was fed to Hendrick directly by the Rockefeller's director, Simon Flexner. These articles, especially 'Conquering Spinal Meningitis: What the Rockefeller Institute Has Done for Children', were written as fables of science, where a dreadful and anthropomorphized disease rips through the communities of the poor and densely populated, killing three-quarters of all the children it touches. Flexner, the doctor hero of this tale, turns to animals in search of both prevention and cure, and finds it in a worthy monkey, indeed, according to Hendrick, 'one of the great monkeys of history'. Thereafter, the protective serum is

---

[52] William Williams Keen, 'Recent Surgical Progress: A Result Chiefly of Experimental Research', *Harper's Monthly*, 118 (1909): 764–73. Re-issued, London: Macmillan, 1909.

[53] W. W. Keen, *Animal Experimentation and Medical Progress* (Boston: Houghton Mifflin, 1914). The volume was introduced by Charles W. Eliot, who highlighted the following in particular: 'One third of the book is devoted to the exposition of the unreasonableness, inaccuracy, and indifference to truth and justice manifested by the antivivisectionists in selecting the premises of their argument against animal experimentation. He points out over and over again that the antivivisectionists would be the cruel people, if they could have their way, cruel to their own kind; and that the surgeons and physiologists, and the men who devoted themselves to medical and surgical research are carrying on the most humane work now done in the world. Dr. Keen thus sets before his readers in a striking way the evil consequences which may flow from the morbid perversion of a humane, kindly, or altruistic sentiment. In this case, the common sense of mankind ought to be able to prevent the victims of a perverted sentiment from doing serious harm to the human race' (xxv), noting that Keen was 'like most good surgeons, a humane and sympathetic man' (xxvi).

[54] We can assume, from later correspondence, that Hendrick had an involved relationship with Flexner, who contributed to a number of Hendrick's other articles on the defense of medical research after he left *McClure's* and went to work for *Harper's* and the *World's Work*. See the series of correspondence from 1913 to 1917 in Reel 52, FA746, Series 1 Simon Flexner Paper; Subseries 1.2 Rockefeller Institute for Medical Research, Simon Flexner Papers (American Philosophical Society), RAC. See also Burton J. Hendrick, 'American Contributions to Medical Science', *Harper's Monthly*, 129 (1914): 25–32.

cultivated in the horse, described as 'Mankind's most patient friend' and, once harvested, delivered unto the sick with remarkable results, not just in the USA but around the civilized world. Children are saved, not only from death, but also largely from the afflictions that often accompanied a recovery from meningitis.[55]

The other article from that year, which focused on work on organ transplantation, introduced the Rockefeller Institute as a place defined by a quest 'not to cure individuals, but to cure humanity'. Its staff worked to give 'freely to mankind' any 'important discovery', without thought of reward beyond the 'satisfaction of having done something worth while'.[56] Such an institution was an emblem of humanity, hope and noble causes. Most importantly here, the work of Alexis Carrel was packaged and presented as something other than a kind of morbid curiosity, or experimental science for its own sake. He had been branded, by the leading American antivivisectionist Caroline Earl White, as 'a thinking machine', in whom 'the finer instincts of humanity are drowned in the one passion for so-called scientific research'.[57] From the outside, an image had been constructed of the Rockefeller as a sort of House of Pain, as in H. G. Wells' *The Island of Doctor Moreau*, which had been published only five years before the foundation of the Institute. That book captures the fire, the anti-civilizational nightmare, of the opponents of vivisection, concerned as they were that the pursuit of knowledge had calcified any semblance of tender mercy in medical researchers, to the point that all ethical barriers to experimentation seemed to be surmountable.[58] Hendrick's summary of Carrel's achievements noted the cross-species transplantation of kidneys, and the successful grafting of one dog's leg onto another – the kinds of practices so easily represented as evidence of monstrosity in medicine – but dismissed any such suggestion of blind callousness: 'what was the miracle of an age of faith', Hendrick reported, 'may become the reality of an age of science'. Indeed Carrel's innovative way of joining severed arteries was described as 'beautiful in its minuteness and its simplicity'.[59] Here was the surgeon as artist and artisan, as well as human benefactor. While Carrel's methods were described in some detail, the narrative packaging made sure to give an overall

---

[55] Burton J. Hendrick, 'Conquering Spinal Meningitis: What the Rockefeller Institute Has Done for Children', *McClure's Magazine*, 32 (1909): 594–604.

[56] Burton J. Hendrick, 'Work at the Rockefeller Institute: The Transplanting of Animal Organs', *McClure's Magazine*, 32 (1909): 367–83.

[57] Quoted in an open letter forwarded to Cannon from Simmons, written by Grace D. Davis, secretary of the Society for the Prevention of Abuse in Animal Experimentation, 12 November 1908, H MS c 40, Folder 333, Box 28, WBCA.

[58] H. G. Wells, *The Island of Doctor Moreau* (London: Heinemann, 1896).

[59] Hendrick, 'Work at the Rockefeller', 370, 371–2.

impression of sensitivity, humane purpose and positive outcomes.[60] The effect was to garner public support for medical science under the banner of the secular miracle, at moments when antivivisectionists threatened to restrict medical science through the law. It made such activities seem like apostasy.

This kind of emplotment also crept into scientific publications.[61] As early as 1908, Cannon had a memorandum sent to the editors of all prominent American medical journals, begging them to 'aid the efforts of the Council by very careful examination of articles submitted to you for publication, with special reference to the use of words likely to cause misapprehension regarding the experience of the animals used for research'. Use of anaesthetics in particular was to be reported explicitly.[62] By 1914, at the behest of Richard Pearce (Professor of Research Medicine at the University of Pennsylvania), the letter was reissued, edited by Pearce, again demanding 'careful editorial scrutiny', but also stressing consent where humans, and especially children, were employed for new methods of diagnosis and treatment, and insisting on an emphasis on the 'practical application' of animal experiments in 'the relief of suffering in man'.[63] Moreover, all of the CDMR's pamphlets, which were issued individually, were originally published in the *Journal of the American Medical Association*, for an essentially professional medical audience, but all of them with due sensitivity to the question of humane purpose (a disease, a surgical problem, public health), humane practice (anaesthetics, chiefly), and humane outcomes (the human

---

[60] Carrel had read *The Island of Doctor Moreau* and had shared it with Dr Howard Lilienthal, who thanked him for it while noting that 'It is certainly a quaint and queer tale'. Doubtless Carrel found amusement in it, even though it helped fuel the tirades against him. Lilienthal to Carrel, 30 April 1908, Folder 18, Box 2, FA208, Series 2: Carrel Files, Theodore Malinin collection of Alexis Carrel and Charles Lindbergh papers, RAC.

[61] Susan Lederer, 'Political Animals: The Shaping of Biomedical Research Literature in Twentieth-Century America', *Isis*, 83 (1992): 61–79, puts a clear emphasis on the editorial oversight and imposition of Francis Peyton Rous at the *Journal of Experimental Medicine* from 1921. I would argue that, with regard to the sore spot of vivisection, medical scientists had been editorially self-conscious ever since Burdon Sanderson et al.'s *Handbook* was published in 1873 without any mention of anaesthetic. The controversy surrounding that omission put scientists on high alert when putting pen to paper. Lederer herself points to the actions of the CDMR in language management in medical journals in *Subjected to Science*, 94.

[62] Quoted in Cannon to Pearce, 25 March 1914, H MS c 40, Folder 358, Box 29, WBCA.

[63] Pearce to Cannon, 24 March 1914, Cannon to Pearce, 25 March 1914, Pearce's loose enclosure with edited text plus Cannon's emendations, H MS c 40, Folder 358, Box 29, WBCA. Pearce had worked under Flexner at U Penn between 1900 and 1903, before directing the Bureau of Pathology of the New York State Board of Health. He was famously tried for cruelty to animals, along with others, in 1914, and acquitted, in an attempt to prosecute vivisectors under existing animal welfare legislation. Pearce's own significant contribution to the defense of research was his five-part article in *Popular Science Monthly*, 80–81 (1912), 'Research in Medicine'.

value of the application of research).[64] Somewhat earlier than this, beginning in 1908 and running throughout 1909, the Committee on Experimental Medicine of the Medical Society of the State of New York had begun issuing its own pamphlets, in runs of 10 000.[65] Clearly, with such numbers there was a hope to reach beyond the medical profession. Cannon himself ordered fifty copies of each of the New York pamphlets, to distribute to the CDMR committee and to the members of the legislative committee overseeing a new antivivisection Bill in the Massachusetts State Legislature.[66] The series combined medical expertise and academic prominence, but the soberly scientific format and writing could serve both communities. Given the large number of physicians (some 700) in the state of New York who had backed the Davis-Lee antivivisection Bill, these essentially academic pamphlets did vital work among the wider medical profession to engage and persuade that medical research was not inhumane and required no external policing.[67]

To some extent, all of this work, scientific and lay, and the images with which this chapter opened, recapitulated an argument that had already been alive for a generation, on both sides of the Atlantic. But something had changed: all strains of philosophical or ideological dogma, such as the Utilitarian slogan of 'the greatest happiness for the greatest number', which had coloured similar debates in England in the 1870s and 1880s, had been ditched in favour of simple stories that comprised a new genre: the modern medical miracle. In the stories and reports that emerged,

---

[64] From the CDMR's inception in 1908 until 1914, it published 27 'Defense of Research' pamphlets, sticking to the general theme of the humanity or mercy of vivisection and, conversely, the ill effects of antivivisection. Representative titles include pamphlet 23, W. B. Cannon, *Animal Experimentation and Its Benefit to Mankind* (Chicago: AMA, 1912), and pamphlet 24, W. W. Keen, *The Influence of Antivivisection on Character* (Chicago: AMA, 1912). Within this general theme, there were, of course, more specific case studies to exemplify the point, such as pamphlet 21, Charles Hunter Dunn, *Animal Experimentation in Relation to Epidemic Cerebrospinal Meningitis* (Chicago: AMA, 1911), and pamphlet 17, Frederick P. Gay, *Immunology: A Medical Science Developed through Animal Experimentation* (Chicago: AMA, 1910).

[65] Lee to Cannon, 29 January 1909, H MS c 40, Folder 339, Box 28, WBCA. A sample of the New York Medical Society's pamphlets includes the following: F. S. Lee, *The Sense of Pain in Man and the Lower Animals* (1908); Simon Flexner, *Animal Experimentation and Infectious Diseases* (1908); James Ewing, *Animal Experimentation and Cancer* (1908); George F. Clover, *Animal Experimentation as Viewed by the Superintendent of a Hospital* (1909); Jacob Gould Schurman [president of Cornell University], *President Schurman on Animal Experimentation* (1909); Charles W. Eliot, *Animal Experimentation as Viewed by Laymen* (1909); Graham Lusk, *Animal Experimentation and Diabetes* (1909); Edward L. Trudeau, *Animal Experimentation and Tuberculosis* (1909); William H. Park, *Animal Experimentation and Diphtheria* (1909); Charles L. Dana, *The Service of Animal Experimentation to the Knowledge and Treatment of Nervous Diseases* (1909).

[66] Cannon to Lee, 30 January 1909, H MS c 40, Folder 339, Box 28, WBCA.

[67] Unti, 'The Doctors Are So Sure', 177.

tendencies towards awe and wonder were tethered by explanation. New knowledge, courtesy of experimentation, supplanted any tendency towards to the magical. There was no mystery or mystique, just openness and the banality of process, of men – almost always men – doing hard bloody work, for the most noble of causes.[68]

Forging Ties

For all that there were genuine medical benefits of animal experimentation to report and detail, the most important thing here was the emplotment of the story of medical research. The plot gave the medical details purpose, and made the researchers into heroes. Perhaps more importantly, the plot did not *require* details. To be sure, details could be summoned if demanded, if the 'usefulness' of experiment had to be demonstrated, but the creation of a new class of American hero required a more simple message. Flexner himself was clear about the reasons for this, telling a hearing on two antivivi-section Bills before the New York Senate Judiciary Committee that no person who was not 'highly qualified' or 'highly trained' in this 'highly specialized' work of animal experimentation could possibly state the purpose or value of any particular experiment. Laboratories were 'places which are really promoting the public good' and it was no use exposing them to people 'who have no knowledge on the subject'.[69] Indeed, on another occasion he explicitly warned against the judgement of 'persons who are not scientifically trained', whose judgements were 'influenced ... by a consideration of emotion and sentiment'.[70] This was a far cry from John Simon's assertion that the lay public was listening and able, readily, to understand. Flexner had

---

[68] On the question of gender, see below. It has been put to me on more than one occasion that, looking back from the 1920s, the trope of the medical miracle was indeed imbued with a kind of magic or mystique, with Julian Huxley's 'Tissue-Culture King' (1926) being an exemplary case in point. A pastiche, in many ways, of Wells' *Island of Doctor Moreau*, Huxley's account of the captured experimental biologists, making immortal tissue cultures, strange creatures, and tampering with genetics, is miraculous only to those native actors who exist in extreme isolation from western science. When another Englishman is captured, all the 'miracles' are explained very clearly as arising out of simple extensions of known procedures. While the research impresses the newcomer compatriot, it does not *surprise* him from a scientific point of view. Indeed, the research is conducted, as with Moreau's, on rational lines to monstrous ends. It may look like a magical process from the outside, but to those who know how the trick is done, there is no need for the suspension of disbelief.

[69] Hearing on Senate Bills 170 and 791 In Re Vivisection before Senate Judiciary Committee, Albany, 24 March 1909, 8–9, Folder 19, Box 2, FA142 Anti-vivisection Activities, RUR, RAC.

[70] Hearing before the Senate Judiciary Committee on Bill to Create a Commission to Investigate Animal Experimentation, Albany, New York, 18 February 1913, Folder 22, Box 2, FA142, Anti-vivisection Activities, RUR, RAC.

cause to be so exclusive. At the end of 1909, the notorious 'Rockefeller Affidavits' – a series of eye-witness accounts of laboratory horrors from former functionary employees at the Rockefeller – were published in the *New York Herald*, to the great dismay of medical scientists in the USA and in Britain, where they were picked up by prominent antivivisectionists. These first-hand accounts were gainsaid by Flexner, but it did not stop them resurfacing, again and again, in subsequent years.[71]

A fine line had to be walked: the public was asked, on the one hand, to trust and believe the medical authorities on the basis that its methods and its production of knowledge could be made plain, through communications in straightforward language, to the non-expert; and on the other hand, the public was asked to mind its own business and let doctors get on with their work because they could not possibly understand what they were doing.

Somewhere in the middle of this apparent paradox was a sweet spot: a place where the public could be satisfied with *enough* information to reassure them that nothing immoral or purposeless was happening in medical laboratories, but not too much to prevent them from reading it, and not too little so as to leave lingering doubts. For example, Jerome Greene at the Rockefeller asked Alexis Carrel for a statement about certain of his experiments in January 1912, in order to be prepared to meet the antivivisectionist onslaught that year. The statement, he exhorted, had to be able to 'be grasped by a layman, showing not only the defects or distortions' of the antivivisectionist position, 'but also the humane and intelligent purpose which actuated' the experimental work in the first place.[72] The medical establishment's core strategy involved packaging medical knowledge into digestible accounts of the moral virtue of experimentation, while preserving the exclusivity of the deep understanding that underlay medical practice (this was supported by targeted lectures at elite and/or academic groups).[73]

---

[71] One of the principal affidavits was by a person Flexner called 'The Kennedy woman', employed as a 'scrubwoman'. Flexner pointed out her hypocrisy – she had once stolen a cat and offered it to the Rockefeller for money; she was reputedly offered $100 by antivivisectionists to tell all – and insisted that it was 'an imposition upon a lay public, · uninformed and properly so of the methods of the hospital operating room, to parade as wanton cruelty when applied to the brute creation the very means which are in daily use to save life and limb in the best hospitals'. Simon Flexner, *The So-Called 'Affidavits Concerning the Atrocities of Vivisection': A Refutation*, pamphlet, reprinted from the *New York Times*, 17 January 1910, Folder 20, Box 2, FA142, Anti-vivisection activities, RUR, RAC. The affidavits were originally published in the *New York Herald*, 27 and 28 December 1909.

[72] Greene to Carrel, 8 January 1912, Folder 9, Box 2, FA208, Series 2: Carrel Files, Theodore Malinin collection of Alexis Carrel and Charles Lindbergh papers, RAC.

[73] Lee, for example, took the train up to Dartmouth to lecture 600 students for an hour on the virtues of vivisection. Lee to Greene, 3 April 1911, Box 2, FA808, Series 2 Business Manager Correspondence, RUR, RAC.

The message, therefore, was one of mercy, or humanity, and of the greatness that inhered in the meek, indefatigable quest for salvation from disease.

The heroic was devoid of the typical drama of derring-do or action, but activated by dogged, hidden, high-minded recluses to save people through new knowledge and the application of new knowledge. As Cannon put it, medical scientists were part of a 'brotherhood of venturesome men' for whom 'the zest of life lies in the discoveries and conquests in the unmapped wilderness'. Men of science were like American pioneers, the spirit of which moved them 'in the search for truth'.[74] The favourable sections of the press agreed entirely. *Collier's*, for example, posited that 'The question of when to use anesthetics must be left to science, since in a small but important fraction of the work drugs must be dispensed with; and it would be fatal to have ignorant outsiders concerned in so critical a decision. Such outsiders are capable of judging sanely neither about the amount of pain involved nor the importance of the knowledge to be obtained'. To stop animal experimentation, or even to interfere with it, would 'take away our strongest weapon' in the fight against so many scourges of humanity.[75]

In order to promote themselves in such a way, experimenters relied on indirect communication with the public. Their heroic example required third parties to put them forward, at arms length from medical science itself. Such distance removed from the public representation of medical science any sense of special pleading. Journalism – the guarantor of honesty in public life, or so some held it up to be – would not bend to medical falsehoods and propaganda. The raking light of the press would editorialize medical science for what it really was.

This is romantic, of course. The parts of the popular press that favoured the medical experimenters were interested in promoting American civilization, to be sure, but they were also horrified by other parts of the popular press that had given up any kind of service to the truth or to editorial ethics. The gutter press commanded an immense readership and undermined public opinion with scurrilous stories and, for want of a better phrase, 'fake news'. *The New York Herald* was, in this period, at the forefront of say-anything populism, and the mainstream press rallied to shout it down. As such, large parts of the press and the medical-science community found they had a mutual interest in one another. Lasting

---

[74] Walter B. Cannon, 'The Ideals of the Man of Science: An Address', printed publication, c. 1913, H MS c 40, Folder 373, Box 30, WBCA. In his memoir, Cannon noted the importance of his ancestry and the traditions it had established in his family. Notably, he was descended from a French Canadian *coureur de bois*. He literally embodied the spirit of the explorer. Walter B. Cannon, *The Way of an Investigator: A Scientist's Experiences in Medical Research* (New York: W. W. Norton, 1945), 11.

[75] 'Vivisection', *Collier's*, 23 January 1909, 6.

relationships were formed that would become the backbone of strategies for the public defence of research. The assistant editor of the *Boston Herald*, for example, told Cannon in 1914 that the paper was 'ready and willing to do whatever it can at all times to help the advance of science and of truth', pointing out along the way that the 'Christian Scientists, the anti-vaccinationists and the whole kit and boodle of freaks have no hesitation in shouting from the house tops', and that it was down to scientists to put their serious voices into the mix.[76] Earlier that same year, Cannon had told the same editor that he was grateful for the *Herald*'s 'admirable support'. One article in particular – 'a gem' – was clipped by Cannon and sent to the *Journal of the American Medical Association*, where it would be 'republished ... and sent all over the country to nearly sixty thousand physicians'.[77] Such was the power of the medical-journalistic relationship.

Most significant of all, perhaps, was the relationship between Flexner and the Rockefeller business managers with the writer and editor Norman Hapgood (1868–1937) and the publications of S. S. McClure. Hapgood was editor at *Collier's* from 1903 until 1913, and provided much favourable content for the defence of medical research, reaching a vast audience with its muckraking exposés. From 1913, *Harper's Weekly* came under the ownership of McClure Publications in New York and quickly adopted a favourable attitude to medical science, under the editorship of Hapgood, who moved there from *Collier's*. *Harper's* was the leading serious newspaper of record in the USA in the years before 1900, commanding a circulation in excess of 100 000, and a readership of perhaps 500 000. Though waning by the time it was sold to McClure, it was still shaped by influential opinion and formative of public opinion on a wealth of issues. *Harper's*, as with *Collier's* in earlier years, was staunchly in favour of the benefits of vivisection, and deferred entirely to the information supplied by medical scientists in order to write pieces in praise of it. This initiative came directly from the editor in chief, in correspondence with Flexner and co. In addition, as we have already seen, the medical establishment had a great friend in *Puck* magazine, which had come out definitively and graphically in favour of vivisection as an act of mercy.

The relationship between the New York doctors in particular and Hapgood is exemplary of the manner in which the medical establishment sought to influence public opinion vicariously, while still being in absolute control of the messaging. We can assume that the relationship was long-running, given the manner of Hapgood's editorializing in *Collier's* and later *Harper's*, but we have good evidence for the level of medical involvement

[76] E. H. Gruening to Cannon, 6 May 1914, H MS c 40, Folder 362, Box 30, WBCA.
[77] Cannon to Gruening, 26 March 1914, H MS c 40, Folder 362, Box 30, WBCA.

in the production of positive press from one series of correspondence in the spring of 1914. It begins with a letter from Hapgood to Flexner, alerting him to an article in *Cosmopolitan*, owned by that date by William Randolph Hearst (1863–1951), written by the arch antivivisectionist Diana Belais, and calling it 'an outrage for them to take part in stirring up this subject again'.[78] While Belais had ranged freely across the well-trodden ground of antivivisectionist argumentation, it was her casual mention of 'thousands of children' who had been 'experimented upon with tuberculin, with vaccines, with syphilitic cultures' that particularly drew ire, for it squarely pointed at the work of Rockefeller scientists and dredged up Noguchi's 1911 experiments trying to find an improved diagnostic test for syphilis once again.[79] Noguchi had used wards of the state – orphans – as part of his human testing of his inert 'luetin' substance, which had previously been tested on animals (and on himself).[80] Privately, Flexner warned off Richard Pearce from 'getting into a controversy in the Cosmopolitan', despite Pearce's eagerness to prepare a 'popular account of animal experimentation'.[81] But Flexner knew there was a case to answer. It was simply better met by professional journalists, with a buffer between public discourse and the experts who would feed it. It is clear from a letter a couple of weeks later from Henry James Jr, the

---

[78] Hapgood to Flexner, 10 March 1914, Folder 4, Box 6, FA142, Anti-vivisection activities, RUR, RAC.

[79] Diana Belais, 'Why Vivisection?', *Cosmopolitan*, 56 (1914): 649–53. The article followed another in the same volume (Ella Wheeler Wilcox, 'Vivisection and Surgery', 572–4), which again dredged up the oft-dismissed Rockefeller affidavits.

[80] Hideyo Noguchi, 'A Cutaneous Reaction in Syphilis', *Journal of Experimental Medicine*, 14 (1911): 557–68. The dubious ethics (and results) of Noguchi's experiments, the antivivisectionist response to them and the Rockefeller's defence of them, are detailed in Lederer, 'Hideyo Noguchi'. The context, historiographically, is on the lack of consent in these clinical experiments. Seen from within its own historical context, however, neither the antivivisectionist attacks on Noguchi nor his colleagues' defence focused *primarily* upon this question, even though it was already an active ethical issue. The antivivisectionist response, and the media event in 1914, focused instead on the spurious claim that medical scientists were actually infecting children with syphilis. The medical response was mainly to issue denials in good faith, as well as pointing to the fact that Noguchi's experiments had proven useful without causing harm. As Lederer details ('Hideyo Noguchi's luetin experiment', 39) the New York Society for the Prevention of Cruelty to Children did raise the issue of consent, but to no avail in legal terms. In purely utilitarian terms, the orthodox moral calculus of the time justified Noguchi's experiments, but the rise of clinical experimentation on humans would lead to retrospective second guessing among laboratory scientists. See the epilogue.

[81] Pearce to Flexner, 18 March 1914, and Flexner to Pearce, 19 March 1914, Flexner Pearce correspondence, pt 2, Reel 88, FA746, Series 1 Simon Flexner Paper; Subseries 1.2 Rockefeller Institute for Medical Research, Simon Flexner Papers (American Philosophical Society), RAC. Pearce would ultimately prepare a piece for the CDMR series of pamphlets published by the AMA: Richard Pearce, *The Charge of 'Human Vivisection' as Presented in Antivivisection Literature* (Chicago: American Medical Association, 1914).

Rockefeller's business manager, that in the interim Hapgood had actually visited the Rockefeller in person, specifically to discuss Frederick Bellamy, who annually stirred up legislative activity in New York. Hapgood wanted to explore the financing of antivivisection and the activity of New York antivivisection societies. James duly supplied him with plenty of information, including correspondence with Cannon.[82] Hapgood also tapped F. S. Lee for more detail, noting his 'impression that Frederick Bellamy is kept going by a fund left by a cat-loving woman who is dead', and Lee duly obliged, picking up Hapgood's forwarded correspondence at his club in Brunswick, Georgia.[83] Lee responded with acerbic wit, detailing the antivivisection activities of Mrs Gazzam, 'a wealthy lady of Cornwall-on-the-Hudson', whom Bellamy represented until her death. After she died, her activism was taken up by a daughter, 'of whose eccentricities strange tales are told', notably concerning her 'original ideas about love' and an entanglement with a 'mind-curist out in California'. In short, Lee painted Bellamy's associations as ludicrous, emotionally imbalanced and dangerously wealthy. He told Hapgood that Bellamy was a 'rather guileless cuss' and thought with 'a proper exercise of sympathy [he] might easily be induced ... to give himself away', encouraging Hapgood to write his story. Lee had, so he told Hapgood, 'no confidence in his [Bellamy's] possession of elevated motives. In fact the more I become acquainted with the antivivisection movement the more I appreciate the unworthiness of it both intellectually and morally'.[84] Hapgood duly obliged the doctors and the Rockefeller manager by keeping them apprised of his progress in writing and prospective publication dates.[85] The work was then handed off, for Hapgood felt his load too heavy.[86]

Over the course of several months, the story grew to become a general denunciation of antivivisection and the role of William Randolph Hearst in spreading its lies in the *American*, *Cosmopolitan*, and elsewhere, through an association with Bellamy. The article was taken on by Katharine Loving Buell, who worked closely with Henry James to produce it. When the article appeared, in May 1914, Buell wrote to James to tell him how pleased Hapgood had been to hear of all of James' hard work on

[82] James to Hapgood, 23 March 1914, Folder 4, Box 6, FA142, Anti-vivisection activities, RUR, RAC.
[83] Hapgood to Lee, 17 March 1914, Folder 17, Box, 1, Lee Papers, Augustus C. Long Health Sciences Library, Columbia University, New York (CU).
[84] Lee to Hapgood, 21 March,1914, Folder 4, Box 6, FA142, Anti-vivisection activities, RUR, RAC.
[85] Hapgood to James, 24 March 1914, Folder 4, Box 6, FA142, Anti-vivisection activities, RUR, RAC.
[86] Hapgood to James, 3 June 1914, Folder 4, Box 6, FA142, Anti-vivisection activities, RUR, RAC.

the article. Buell added: 'I could never have produced a respectable piece of work in so short a time if it had not been for the trouble that you took to read copy for me and to write up the technical points'.[87] In sum, the business manager of the Rockefeller Institute was the de facto ghost writer of a major editorial in the popular press that denounced Hearst and the antivivisectionists.

The article itself, which appeared under the title, 'A Campaign of Lies', came replete with illustrations, including one of the *American's* most scurrilous headlines, claiming that the Rockefeller's Dr Noguchi had experimented on 1000 babies.[88] Such stories were dismissed as harmful trash, appealing 'to the passions of an unenlightened class'. The *Cosmopolitan* articles were dismissed has having been penned by 'well-meaning sentimentalists' (this despite the editorial note that topped Belais' article that explicitly foregrounded the 'more important reasons' for antivivisection, which had 'no foundation in mere sentiment').[89] Hearst's readers in general were described as 'poor and ignorant ... afraid of authority wherever they find it'. Yet ultimately it was the poor and ignorant, so the argument went, who suffered as a result of all this noise. Such was the article's climax, a recapitulation of the core argument of medical science: vivisectors were 'busy men of science who are working hard for the benefit of humanity'. The antivivisectionist media campaigns, conversely, caused 'innocent children and helpless sick people' to lose their lives. Unsurprisingly, given the amount of material put into such a piece, from James, Cannon and Lee, it concluded with the standard negotiation of the terms of humanitarianism.[90]

After the article was published the relationship with Buell only deepened, with Hapgood and James ensuring that Buell could visit the Rockefeller laboratories and become even better acquainted with them.[91] Doubtless, it was considered an immense advantage to have the position of medical science conveyed to the public through a female voice.

Hysteria

It had never been lost on those at the forefront of the defence of research that antivivisectionist activity was almost universally understood to be a female predilection, seen respectively as an expression of political awakening and empowerment among women of a like mind, and as

[87] Buell to James, 5 June 1914, Folder 4, Box 6, FA142, Anti-vivisection activities, RUR, RAC.
[88] Katharine Loving Buell, 'A Campaign of Lies', *Harper's Weekly*, 16 May 1914, 13–17.
[89] Belais, 'Why Vivisection?', 649.   [90] Buell, 'A Campaign of Lies', 15.
[91] James to Hapgood, 9 June 1914, Folder 4, Box 6, FA142, Anti-vivisection activities, RUR, RAC.

evidence of sentimentality and emotional unfitness for public life – hysteria, in short – on the part of their opponents. That the medical establishment saw in such women a derogation of femininity was clear. Cannon wrote Paget in 1909 to compare Dr William Williams Keen, a 'thoroughly charming gentleman', with the 'very attractive young woman appealing for legislation' at a hearing in Pennsylvania who had 'called him a hyena!' It was, implicitly, a betrayal of her looks to speak so ill of the refined.[92] In F. S. Lee's estimation, the 'antivivisection view is psychologically of great interest. It rests on a low intellectual and ethical level, and exhibits in an elemental simplicity the qualities and power of emotion. Its abnormal sympathy for animals blinds its possessor to a normal sympathy for human beings'. This could only be a reflection on the weak emotional constitution of women, or else of the effeminate constitution of antivivisectionists who happened to be men. Antivivisectionists were, according to Lee, 'fighting a monster that does not exist'.[93]

The opponents of antivivisection were, conversely, generally understood to be men of science, and their maleness was indeed thought to supply an air of rational coolness, often implicitly, but not uncommonly by explicit argument.[94] Women, therefore, were both seen as the principal enemies of medical research, as well as being the principal target of medical strategies of representation.

These strategies took a number of forms. Direct engagement in person was common. For example, Charles W. Eliot, who until 1909 was the president of Harvard University, had preached with Cannon on the virtues of animal experimentation to 700 society women of the future by capturing them at a formative time in the course of their studies at Wellesley College.[95] Flexner himself had lectured before the Women's League in 1908, even carrying a vote on the virtues of vivisection.[96] In 1912, Lee lectured to 150 members of the New York League of Unitarian

---

[92] Cannon to Paget, 15 March 1909, H MS c 40, Folder 340, Box 28, WBCA.

[93] F. S. Lee, 'The Role of Experiment in Medicine: The Public and the Medical Profession', in *Scientific Features of Modern Medicine* (New York: Columbia University Press, 1911), 161–2.

[94] That most medical scientists were, in fact, men, distinctly overshadows the significant pioneering presence of female researchers whose activities were lost – at least to the lay public – in the noise of a strictly gendered representational tactic. There were occasional attempts to give female voices within medical science a voice (see below), but these were exceptional. In any case, prior to the First World War, when this study ends, medical science at an institutional level can certainly be accurately described as a male domain. See Elizabeth Hanson, 'Women Scientists at the Rockefeller Institute, 1901–1940', in Stapleton, *Creating a Tradition*, 211–25.

[95] Cannon to Greene, 1 March 1911, Folder Cannon, Walter b, Box 1, FA872, Correspondence and biography, RUR, RAC.

[96] Welch to Flexner, 19 May 1908, Reel 7, FA746, Series 1 Simon Flexner Paper; Subseries 1.1 Personal Papers, Simon Flexner Papers (American Philosophical Society), RAC.

Women in Brooklyn (an event crashed by a Philadelphia antivivisection society, much to Lee's chagrin).[97]

In 1914, Richard Pearce wrote to Frederick R. Green, who headed the AMA Council on Health and Public Instruction, recommending a man be found to summarize two articles on war surgery for the CDMR series. On reflection, Pearce wondered whether the author of one of those articles, Dr Alice Hamilton (1869–1970), might 'be the best person to write' such a piece. After all, 'an article by a woman ... would have a distinct value', if one considered the fact that 'most of our opponents are women'.[98] Pearce went further, echoing the sentiments of the English Research Defence Society, telling Flexner in 1914 that 'I am making a move now to start a Women's League for the Protection of Scientific Research – get as many mothers as possible into it, and keep women doctors and doctor's [sic] wives in the back ground', presumably to offer the most convincing lay support possible.[99]

Despite all these examples of positive attempts to engage women and directly appeal to them to support medical research, the overwhelming attitude of the medical establishment was decidedly anti-women, or at the very least suspicion of women's capacity to understand or tolerate vivisection. In the margin of Pearce's letter suggesting a women's league, Flexner had scrawled 'Is this wise?' with the rhetorical implication that indeed it was not.[100] Pearce himself had acknowledged that the enemy was characteristically female, and had relayed a typical encounter at an antivivisectionist meeting in Atlantic City, where a 'Miss or Mrs. Crane-Couch' was horrified to have Pearce even sit next to her. She 'pulled aside her skirts and said, "The idea of you sitting beside me, I wouldn't sit beside you for anything in the world"'. Pearce reported that she then 'took a seat two chairs away and during the half hour discussion cursed and berated me continually'.[101] But Pearce had not written merely to complain, but to share intelligence. It was fairly common for prominent medical scientists to inform each other about the women they encountered. Pearce summed up the problem to Green as follows: 'The really rabid members [of the human societies] are limited to a comparatively small group of women'.[102] The epithet 'rabid' was by no

---

[97] Lee to Greene, 8 April 1912, Folder 6, Box 6, FA142, Anti-vivisection activities, RUR, RAC.

[98] Pearce to Green, 9 October 1914, H MS c 40, Folder 359, Box 29, WBCA; Pearce to Cannon, 26 October 1914, H MS c 40, Folder 359, Box 29, WBCA.

[99] Pearce to Flexner, 21 April 1914, Folder 7, Box 6, FA142, Anti-vivisection activities, RUR, RAC.

[100] Pearce to Flexner, 21 April 1914, Folder 7, Box 6, FA142, Anti-vivisection activities, RUR, RAC.

[101] Pearce to Cannon, 9 October 1914, H MS c 40, Folder 359, Box 29, WBCA.

[102] Pearce to Green, 9 October 1914, H MS c 40, Folder 359, Box 29, WBCA.

means unusual, and with no lack of irony compared the complainants against vivisection to diseased dogs. When one Sarah Cleghorn wrote to the Rockefeller to request a visit – a tour of all the facilities and to see the animals – giving as a reference Dr Allen Starr (1854–1932) to confirm that she was a 'mature and reliable person', Henry James Jr sought out that reference and received a reply that Cleghorn was a 'cranky little old spinster from Vermont', who was 'daft on the subject of anti-vivisection'. Under those circumstances, James initially thought it best simply not to answer her letter.[103] Ultimately, he did so, but he did so with a certain amount of scorn: 'If I am not mistaken you are quite actively interested in the anti-vivisectionist agitation and ... I infer that it is with the purpose of ascertaining whether our experiments are carried on in a manner that would commend itself to your judgement that you wish to visit the laboratories'. James saw no reason to 'multiply interruptions' to the Rockefeller's work, 'in order to satisfy the curiosity or doubts of persons without knowledge to form a competent judgement of the purposes, methods and conduct of animal experimentation, and who have already announced a pre-judgement against the value and propriety of experimental research'.[104]

Just as the press reflected the attitudes of the medical establishment with regard to their other strategies, so it seems reasonable to judge that the press's condemnation of female activism fairly echoed that of medical science itself. In the early days of the CDMR, *Collier's* published an essay by Frederick Peterson, 'A Nerve Specialist to His Patients: To a Woman Who is Unhappy About Vivisection', in which the generic ignorant complainant against medical science was everywoman. It pointed out a series of hypocrisies, from the unthinking wearing of fur and the consumption of flesh, to the docking of horses and the trimming of dogs' ears. It demanded that she 'read widely ... before adopting a conclusion', while lauding the 'higher order of man ... supermen indeed', who 'sacrifice their time for the good of others', in order to make 'glorious discoveries' that 'they give to humanity free of charge with all speed': the 'searchers for the cause and cure of disease' by animal experimentation.[105] And early in 1910 – the year

---

[103] Cleghorn to Rockefeller directors, 17 December 1915, Folder 2, Box 6, FA142, Anti-vivisection activities, RUR, RAC; Memorandum, 27 December 1915, Folder 2, Box 6, FA142, Anti-vivisection activities, RUR, RAC.

[104] James to Cleghorn, 15 January 1916, Folder 2, Box 6, FA142, Anti-vivisection activities, RUR, RAC. Curiously, Walter Cannon did give Cleghorn a tour of the laboratories at Harvard, and he told Richard Pearce that some balance had to be struck between allowing visitors and stopping short of an 'open door' that would admit 'every wild and unbalanced person'. Cannon to Pearce, 10 July 1916, Folder 7, Box 6, FA142, Anti-vivisection activities, RUR, RAC.

[105] Frederick Peterson, 'A Nerve Specialist to His Patients: To a Woman Who Is Unhappy about Vivisection', *Collier's*, 28 November 1908, 28–9.

of the Rockefeller affidavits – *Collier's* ran a story glorying in the removal of the Brown Dog statue in Battersea, London, but took the opportunity to bemoan the American antivivisectionists under the heading 'Hysteria'. Beware the interference of the 'cat-loving woman', it warned, decrying the 'spirit of sentimentality based on ignorance' that defined the protest movement. It branded antivivisectionists 'highly wrought sentimentalists … enthusiastic and uninformed'. Why, it mused, should Dr Flexner be told 'just what he may do by a policeman and a lady'?[106]

Perhaps there is no more telling account of the gendering of this debate than that depicted in the images with which this chapter opened. Femininity, across the three Crawford cartoons, is understood as hypocritical, sentimental, ignorant, hysterical and noisy (in the figure of the antivivisectionist), or else frail and vulnerable (in the figure of the poor and sick).

Negotiating Mercy

The new physiological, immunological and surgical knowledges being produced at the Rockefeller, Columbia, Johns Hopkins, Harvard and elsewhere were products of experimental medicine as an emotional practice – a lived experience of humanitarianism – and therefore those knowledges were not merely 'inflected' by the emotions of their producers, but represented a direct expression of the emotions of those who produced them.

There is an addendum to this, concerning the state of knowledge *about* knowledge. While I would argue strongly that the procedural activities of medical scientists were construed as compassionate activities, and the knowledge produced was a kind of humane knowledge, those practices were essentially private, the knowledge esoteric and accessible only to specialists, until all of it had been packaged and translated for a lay audience. This making public went beyond the traditional realms of scientific publishing and knowledge sharing (though it also included these things), for science itself was at stake in the public sphere. The antivivisection movement, especially in New York, was populist, unafraid of libel, and willing to say anything about medical scientists in the pages of the *New York Herald* so as to hold up laboratories as houses of horrors to the world, ghastly emblems of the rot in civilization being nurtured by men of great wealth and great influence. What the men of the Rockefeller and other research laboratories did, therefore, was a matter of public interest, and those men worked hard to control the messaging in the popular press for a lay audience.

In their own writings, therefore, as well as in the writings of journalist allies, experimentalists were portrayed as ingenious, indefatigable and

---

[106] 'Hysteria', *Collier's*, 22 January 1910, 8.

humane. Such figures of laboratory humanity were duly introduced to the lay public on the understanding that the value of experimental medicine – the wealth of private funding notwithstanding – hinged on public estimation of its moral value. If the ends of experimentation could not be justified by the means – if this high age of medical *progress*, as it was spun, was built upon a foundation of inhumanity and outright cruelty – then the gains were outweighed by the risks to civilization in general. Under the careful control of men like Cannon, Lee and Flexner, as well as the Rockefeller's astonishingly active business managers, the compassionate impetus and the humanitarian application of all this work was highlighted in the press, feeding back ultimately on scientists themselves to be experienced as confirmation of humanitarianism on a higher plane to anything accessible by the public directly. As Cannon put it, antivivisectionists were 'unacquainted with the problems and methods of medical research' and therefore 'restrict their humanity to the welfare of laboratory animals'. By contrast, the medical profession, 'realizing that more power to fight disease can only come from more knowledge, trusts the deeper humanity of the laboratory-workers who are seeking that knowledge'.[107] Similarly, Lee wrote that biological and medical research 'has demonstrated that it is humanitarian in the highest degree', importantly, for the purposes of my argument, 'both in method and in achievement'. It was, he said, in the interest of a 'broad humanitarianism' that men of medicine and 'the public outside of the medical circle' should 'jealously guard the freedom of scientific experimentation'.[108] Welch had announced to the American Association for the Advancement of Science in December 1907 that the 'agitation for the prohibition of experiments on animals, conducted under the guise of an humane purpose, is fundamentally inhuman, for if it were to succeed the best hopes of humanity for further escape from physical suffering and disease would be destroyed'.[109] It was a remarkably consistent message, endlessly repeated and ceaselessly employed as a slogan for the lay public to digest. Not for nothing did all of the pamphlets issued under the auspices of the Council for the Defense of Medical Research boast Charles W. Eliot's refrain on the front page: 'The humanity which would prevent human suffering is a deeper and truer humanity than the humanity which would save pain or death to animals'.[110]

---

[107] Cannon, 'Medical Control of Vivisection', 821.
[108] Lee, 'Role of Experiment', 162–3.
[109] William Henry Welch, 'The Interdependence of Medicine and Other Sciences of Nature', in *Papers and Addresses* (Baltimore: Johns Hopkins University Press, 1920), 3:344.
[110] The quote was widely peddled. *Collier's* published it in early 1909, having previously praised the knowledge acquired by 'merciful vivisection'. See the issues for 19 December 1908 and 23 January 1909. It originated in Eliot's 1900 remonstrance before the State Legislature of Massachusetts concerning a bill to restrict vivisection and was presented again before another bill in 1901. See Chapter 3.

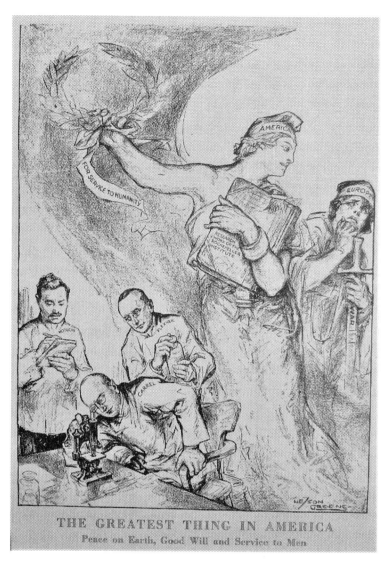

Figure 5.3 'The Greatest Thing in America', *Puck*, 1914.

There is nothing distinctively American about the kind of humanity envisaged as the deepest and truest by Eliot and his medical friends. The line might easily have been uttered in England in the 1870s. Indeed, the entanglement of European and American experiences with antivivisection, and especially the importance of British experience of defending research, suggests a sort of scientific internationalism, defined precisely by its humane purposes, practices and applications. Then again, I do want to suggest that, by the time the Americans became organized and effectively mobilized against antivivisection activism, there was something distinctly American about it. British experience was often used as an example of what to avoid, both in terms of legislation and in terms of the influence of the medical community on public opinion. Whereas Paget in London had sought out lay women and clerics, the Americans resisted any such lay involvement until well after the war. The Americans had to face legislative threats on many fronts, in different states, which rapidly gave them a great experience in dealing with ethical questions about vivisection insofar as they pertained to the law. The British had never had such riches of rehearsal. Moreover, the American medical establishment's engagement with the press, directly at times, but often subtly and in the background, was far in advance of the kind of manipulations of public opinion in Britain. As such, the genre of the medical miracle and of the doctor as merciful hero was perfected in America, and tailored to American middle-class sensibilities in the respectable press.

The distance that had opened up between Britain and America is perhaps best encapsulated in the above image, with which this chapter concludes. It comes, once again, from *Puck*, that long-time ally of medical science. Once more, the artist faithfully depicted the position that American medical scientists had taken up (Figure 5.3). This image is from 1914, shortly after the outbreak of war. Europe, cowed by the nerve-shattering experience of combat, falls in behind the reassuring presence of America, topped with a liberty cap, proudly proclaiming the Rockefeller Institute to be the 'Greatest Thing in America' and donning its three principal scientists, Flexner, Noguchi and Carrel – captured in the process of knowledge production – with a laurel for 'service to humanity'. This notion of service, itself a form of humanitarianism, is intermixed with an idea of 'good will' and 'peace' that is emphatically emblemized by the American melting pot. The accompanying text with this image proudly proclaims that through the spirit of its 'mixed population' working for a common cause, America was bringing home to 'bloody Europe' 'the real lesson of humanity'.[111] Vivisection, as a practice of mercy, had become emblematic of what was good about American society in general, in contradistinction to those bloodthirsty countries across the Atlantic.

---

[111] *Puck*, 76:1971 (12 December 1914).

Epilogue: Humanity and Human Experimentation

The strategic defence of experimental medicine, through professions of humanity that described, in turn, a practice of a self-proclaimed humanitarian professionalism, was a success before the outbreak of war in 1914. On both sides of the Atlantic, the medical establishment had successfully negotiated the antivivisection challenge, through a variety of means: legislative, representational, political, rhetorical. They had, having first entangled themselves in a legislative compromise, beaten the antivivisectionists in terms of organization, in terms of fund-raising, and in terms of authority and influence. They had beaten them through well coordinated transatlantic networks, mastering the control of information and the optics of research. They had beaten them through the tacit control of legislative interventions and processes, exerting a governmental style that was often subtle, sometimes public but often hidden, and always weighted with professional and cultural capital and authority. Most importantly, they had come to practice an experimental discipline with a full conviction that it was humane, that it had the elimination of suffering as its primary end, with the production of knowledge as the means. Humanity had come to be practised with anaesthesia and scalpel. However alien that may seem or sound, its truth is scarcely avoidable. To reclaim it is to recover the medical establishment from a cynical historiographical gaze. Their political and rhetorical manoeuvres were not merely self-serving and practically expedient, but effected in the service of a professional practice that was coded as humane. Such is the overriding argument of this book. A number of ethical tipping points, however, threatened what had become, by 1914, a medical, social and civilizational orthodoxy. Many historiographical threads begin with the First World War. But this is where the thread of this story begins to unravel.

Homo *In Vitro*

When we last met Alexis Carrel it was Carrel the surgeon, whose experimental techniques had won him the Nobel Prize; Carrel the tireless worker; Carrel the miracle maker. But Carrel's attention had been diverted to new experimental possibilities that re-imagined research on the living being, re-conceptualizing life, and, with it, pain, ethics and death. Carrel ushered in the possibility of both the immortal and the post-human. With the promise of tissue-culture methods, life could be studied at the cellular level, with cultures kept alive, in theory, indefinitely. Carrel was not the only one, of course, but the story of the development of tissue-culture research is well known, and not for me to re-tell here. It is only necessary to signal the importance, given the narrative and argument of this book, of the shifting of experimental research on the living to experimental research on life *in vitro*.

While tissue-culture research was only one strand of experimental work, and vivisection in a more traditional manner continued throughout the twentieth century, life in a glass did present an opportunity to say that the 'life' under study was authentically *living* but no longer animal. The logical extension, when culturing human cells, was to say that these human cells lived but were no longer human, in any meaningful sense of the word. Yet human cell cultures promised a massive new production of knowledge about, and applications for, human biology. They were the realization of the animal and the human machine with the *Geist* extracted, the reduction of biological matter to its automatic processes, devoid of consciousness, unsusceptible to suffering, pain or fear. This was life reconceived as unending, neutral, ethically exempt from all of the considerations that had activated opposition to animal experimentation up to that point. New ethical objections would emerge, for tissue culture threatened the very sanctity of life, of the boundaries of the individual, considered as a temporally bound existence attached to subjective experience. Whereas vivisectionists had been accused of abandoning religious conceptions of compassion for a hardened pursuit of knowledge activated by unimpeded curiosity, researchers using tissue culture to examine and manipulate life at the cellular level were playing God. In a manner far less crude than the monstrous creations of Dr Frankenstein, the tissue-culture kings might have been seen to be fabricating life that was human but not *human enough*, in their own eyes, to check their ambitions. While on the one hand it seemed to release research from its ethical constraints, on the other hand it seemed to risk the sanctity and the mystery of life itself. In a post-human world, the whole notion of life and its plasticity was in the balance. The mad-scientist genre thus took a new turn.[1]

---

[1] The exemplar here is the short story by Julian Huxley, 'The Tissue-Culture King', *Cornhill Magazine*, new series 60 (1926): 422–58. For the best account of the rise of tissue culture, the role of Alexis Carrel, and the ethical implications of this turn, see Landecker, *Culturing*

Homo *In Vivo*

George Washington Crile had been exemplary of laboratory humanitarianism in the years prior to the First World War. His work was proof positive of the notion that experiments on animals yielded positive benefits for humans as the research was applied in the world. Yet Crile was frustrated. The laboratory, for all its advantages, and the claims of physiologists notwithstanding, was limited. What was required was experimentation on humans, on a human scale. It was, in peace times, the place to which experiment feared to tread. Indeed, the entire defence of research had been undergirded by an implicit understanding that research on humans was not necessary because of the animal analogue, the usefulness of which was underwritten by an evolutionary view of physiological similarity across species. With the rise of tissue-culture techniques after 1910, even human elements seemed to be within reach, without disturbing the ethical sanctity of the human body itself. And where apparently rogue or over-zealous scientists had overstepped in the realm of human experimentation, the medical community at large had, for a generation, condemned them fiercely, while re-stating their own commitment to laboratory procedures. The war against antivivisection was being won on these terms, though the times and the ethics were increasing in complexity.

The outbreak of war in Europe changed the way that medical science justified itself in experimental terms, bifurcating the community along human and animal lines. On the one hand, the war was the ultimate justification, in the face of antivivisectionist activity, for the pursuit of experimental work in the laboratory. Walter Cannon wrote to Richard Pearce in January 1915, suggesting that the physiological wars were over, or at the least, almost so:

Apparently in the presence of the enormous catastrophe in Europe where nations are thinking that the sacrifice of human life for national welfare is fully justified, the 'Antis' find some difficulty in convincing people that it is wicked to use the liver of a relatively small number of lower animals for the welfare of all mankind as well as the animals themselves. Certainly in all my experience the clippings which mark the interest in the anti-vivisection propaganda have never been so few at this time of the year.[2]

When agitation did threaten, as with new antivivisection Bills in California in 1915 and New York in 1916, both the establishment and their political allies, could waive them away with something like

---

Life, 68–92. Landecker particularly marks Carrel's return from service in the war as a moment when his work shifted from surgery to culturing cells (82).

[2] Cannon to Pearce, 9 January 1915, H MS c 40, Folder 359, Box 29, WBCA.

nonchalance. New York Senator J. Henry Walters wrote to Flexner in February 1918 that he had 'a large supply of opiates and anaesthetics at hand; each clerk has a hypodermic syringe with gallon capacity. Through the painless process that will not annoy the hysterical short haired woman and long haired man the Bills will be quietly laid away'.[3] By 1918, Stephen Paget could tell Simon Flexner that, in England at least, 'The anti-vivisection people over here have rather been thrown out of work by the War'.[4] The oft-stated claim that science could diminish human suffering was, in the context of war, of more acutely expedient use. Whole polities came to hope it were true, in the face of a magnitude of suffering never before witnessed.

For Crile, and others, another possibility presented itself. The war itself was a giant uncontrolled experiment on human pain and suffering, carried out by those whose interests seemed to be to heighten the anguish, rather than to ameliorate it. Crile described what happened to Belgians at the hands of German soldiers as the 'vivisection of Belgium': a 'giant experiment that inflicted physiological damage on the whole population, damage of phylogenetic proportions that upended long-established population-wide norms, even affecting "action patterns in the brains of children"'.[5] The upshot was an opportunity: human subjects, ripe for the experimental trial of new surgical techniques and the exploration of new physiological ideas, were being presented to the medical community on a massive scale. There was, in peacetime, 'no opportunity for the study of human material' concerning the 'effects of fear and exhaustion', but the war made 'such opportunities ... abundant'. Human experimentation, for Crile, had been transformed in the mud of France from an ethical quagmire to be left alone, to a moral imperative and a career opportunity to be seized.[6]

Geroulanos and Meyers point to a generational schism in the world of experimental medicine at this point, with the elder statesman Crile feeling constrained by laboratory limitations. They note that while 'Crile wrote scathingly about the impotence of the laboratory-dwelling physiologist lost in his experimental preoccupations', those physiologists returned 'the compliment by brushing Crile aside as obsolete: they needed and engaged

[3] Walters to Flexner, 23 February 1916, Lee Papers, Box 5, Folder 15. Augustus C. Long Health Sciences Library, Columbia University, New York (CU).
[4] Paget to Flexner, 25 July 1918, Flexner Paget correspondence, Reel 86, FA746, Series 1 Simon Flexner Paper; Subseries 1.2 Rockefeller Institute for Medical Research, Simon Flexner Papers (American Philosophical Society), RAC.
[5] Quoted in Stefanos Geroulanos and Todd Meyers, *The Human Body in the Age of Catastrophe: Brittleness, Integration, Science, and the Great War* (Chicago: University of Chicago Press, 2018), 37.
[6] Geroulanos and Meyers, *Human Body*, 37.

with human clinical material at length and with resolution'.[7] While the split marked a stark divergence at its extreme ends, for many medical scientists the reality of the human bodily wreckage of warfare and the prevailing laboratory impetus became entangled. Experiment remained the order of the day, whether in the laboratory or the clinic, but the shift in medical focus sent the issue of antivivisection rather into the shadows. From the outside of medical science, from the point of view of politicians and lay public opinion, there was less justification than ever for standing in the way of science and its ameliorative initiatives. The war would cement the idea that medical scientists were heroes, aided in large part by their own self-adulation.

War also shifted the ground of experiment inexorably towards the human itself. The political reality that emerged after it, and the increasing extent to which national governments co-opted scientific research under secretive and ultimately military ends, meant that, all the arguments against it notwithstanding, experimental medicine significantly shifted its gaze from the animal to the human. Not only did this betray two generations of fierce rhetoric from within the medical establishment about the intrinsic humanity of medical research, which lent itself all too readily to the logic of military research into the doing of harm, it also undermined other key arguments. Medical scientists had claimed time and again that animal experimentation was not a gateway to human experimentation, but there can be no question that two generations' worth of lessons in physiology, bacteriology, toxicology and so on were directly applied to experiments on humans. Second, the medical establishment had claimed, repeatedly, that their laboratories were open and that admission would be granted to any interested and open-minded party. While what went on there was beyond the ken of the average layperson, medical researchers had never shied away from the thought of demonstrating the humane conditions of their laboratories. As experimental work became a matter of national security it disappeared into a realm of secrecy. The doors were categorically closed. Moreover, there was not even any public knowledge that human experimentation was being carried out.

The history of experimentation on humans in the twentieth century has been told and remains in the process of telling.[8] While much focus has been

---

[7] Geroulanos and Meyers, *Human Body*, 33.

[8] The historiography here is huge, so I suggest the following as a good representative sample: Jordan Goodman and Anthony McElligot, eds, *Useful Bodies: Humans in the Service of Medical Science in the Twentieth Century* (Baltimore: Johns Hopkins University Press, 2003); Ulf Schmidt, *Secret Science: A Century of Poison Warfare and Human Experiments* (Oxford: Oxford University Press, 2015); Ulf Schmidt and A. Frewer, eds, *History and Theory of Human Experimentation: The Declaration of Helsinki and Modern Medical Ethics* (Stuttgart: Franz Steiner, 2007); Lederer, *Subjected to Science*; Gere, *Pain,*

on the case of Germans, for reasons that are all too obvious, all the countries under examination here also engaged in secretive programmes of human experimentation in the context of military research. While there are outliers in the period of study covered by this book, for the most part the threat of human vivisection or human experimentation was not realized prior to 1914. When it did happen, the medical-scientific community tended to condemn it, while sticking to their guns that they were the best judges of what was ethical and what was not. But such arguments would become increasingly difficult.

The Human Experimental Animal

Throughout the years between the 1870s and the First World War, there had been fears among antivivisectionists about experiments on humans. Such fears dominate the narrative of Coral Lansbury's *Old Brown Dog*, and might be thought of as a leitmotiv of the antivivisection movement. The practice of vivisection, so it was claimed, calcified the hearts of medical experimenters, whose attentions would soon turn to more directly relevant objects of study. If animal analogues were useful for the production of knowledge, how much more useful might human bodies be, for men inured to the commission of pain and the spilling of blood? The medical establishment spent much of the period not simply denying specific charges of human experimentation, but denying that this would *ever* form a functional or definitive part of medical science. The defence of vivisection was predicated, above all else, upon its wondrous capacity to produce knowledge for human benefit without any human cost. Scientists might experiment upon themselves, as was their right, but the population had no need to fear for their own health and safety at the hands of medical researchers.

The enormous problem that plagued the strategic defence of medical research was that this seemed, to some extent, to be untrue. By and large, medical research followed through on the conviction that the bodies of animals were good enough, but outlying cases of experimental misadventure, where ambition outstripped ethical concern, did crop up. The reality of their existence, which was usually further distorted by antivivisectionist narratives, was sufficient to keep alive the spectre of human experimentation. It did not matter where these experiments took place. Isolated examples served the antivivisection community in an international context.

Pleasure; Rebecca Lemov, *World as Laboratory: Experiments with Mice, Mazes, and Men* (New York: Hill and Wang, 2006).

One such case was that of Albert Neisser (1855–1916), dermatologist and venerealogist at the University of Breslau. His 1892 experiments with syphilis on nine unwitting prostitutes, some of them minors, became a media event in 1899, after his own reports of the experiments were picked up and spun by antivivisectionists in Munich. Neisser had injected his subjects, without their knowledge, with blood serum extracted from syphilis patients. The intent was to vaccinate, using a cell-free serum, but four of Neisser's patients contracted the disease. For the antivivisectionists, there was no doubt that Neisser had given them the disease, though it is not unlikely that they had contracted it by other means. Nonetheless, the lack of consent in his experimental subjects, and the lack of knowledge that, as patients, they were experimental subjects at all, caused a wave of outcry that brought governmental scrutiny to experimental practices in Germany, and fuelled antivivisectionist discourse about the sinister motives of medical researchers.

The result of Neisser's case was the introduction, in Prussia, of formal protections. As Andreas-Holger Maehle has observed, these protections were not as extensive as they might have been, and still left experimental interventions carried out under a therapeutic umbrella untouched. But they did lay down a formal principle of consent – an acknowledgement that human experimentation was likely to be desirable for medical research – and placed limitations on its extent. Neisser had been punished and fined by the Royal Disciplinary Court for Civil Servants. The Prussian Diet had condemned these kinds of medical experiments and, by the end of 1900, the Prussian Minister for Religious, Educational and Medical Affairs had issued formal instructions that required patients to be informed about the potential risks of what was to be done to them, and to seek their formal consent. Experimentation on children was absolutely prohibited.[9]

Cases such as Neisser's presented a serious problem to the medical establishment. They made inroads into the public sense of trust in the humane professions of experimenters, undermining both their rhetorical position and the honest convictions that supported it. Moreover, while the

---

[9] Andreas-Holger Maehle, *Doctors, Honour and the Law: Medical Ethics in Imperial Germany* (Houndmills, UK: Palgrave, 2009), 82–3. For this case and its broader context, see Lutz Sauerteig, 'Ethische Richtlinien, Patientenrechte and ärztliches Verhalten bei der Arzneimittelerprobung (1892–1931)', *Medizinhistorisches Journal*, 35 (2000): 303–34. For a discussion of clinical experimentation represented as therapeutic medicine, see Christoph Gradmann, '"It Seemed about Time to Try One of Those Modern Medicines": Animal and Human Experimentation in the Chemotherapy of Sleeping Sickness 1905–1908', in *Twentieth Century Ethics of Human Subjects Research: Historical Perspectives on Values, Practices, and Regulations*, ed. Volker Roelcke (Stuttgart: Franz Steiner, 2004).

introduction of regulations concerning ethical safeguards, informed consent and so on might seem like progressive steps in the history of medical ethics, they worked against the principles that medical scientists had been desperately trying to uphold, namely that doctors could be *trusted* to work in the best interests of society, without governmental oversight or intervention. The perceived need for legal regulation or prohibition carried the implication that without such regulation doctors would not know the limits of what was ethically acceptable. The specific professional and legal context of Prussia, or of Germany per se, was not accounted for in the transmission of information from one context of antivivisection to another.

The political fall out of Neisser's case was picked up in London, via a Reuters telegram printed in the *London Daily Chronicle*, and this was soon reproduced in the USA. The American Humane Association's pamphlet, *Human Vivisection: A Statement and an Inquiry*, was reissued with an insert quoting the Reuter's dispatch in full, framing rhetorical arguments that forecast human vivisection with the new empirical proofs thereof. The Reuter's report included Rudolf Virchow's statement protesting that while '*there was no justification for the Breslau experiments*', restrictions on research should be limited so as not to 'close the door altogether to experiments', especially 'rational experiments'.[10] That view would prevail, of course, but it could easily be presented as a hollow appeal to a form of reason that had lost its grip on humanity. Such views were extended by works such as Albert Moll's *Ärztliche Ethik* (1902), which summarized some 600 cases of experimentation on humans drawn from international medical literature. As Moll put it:

> I have observed with increasing surprise that certain medics, obsessed by a kind of research mania, have ignored the areas of law and morality in a most problematic manner. For them, the freedom of research goes so far that it destroys any consideration for others. The borderline between human and animal is blurred for them. The unfortunate sick person that has entrusted herself to their treatment is shamefully betrayed by them, their trust is betrayed, and the human being degraded to a guinea pig. Some of these cases have happened in clinics whose directors can't talk enough about 'humanitarianism', so that one might almost regard them as specialists in humanitarianism. There seem to be no national or political borders for this kind of aberration.[11]

Clearly, the medical establishment had successfully broadcast its commitment to humanity, but remained unable to trust members of its own community not to cause outrage.

---

[10] American Humane Association, *Human Vivisection: A Statement and an Inquiry*, 3rd edn (1900).
[11] Quoted in Maehle, *Doctors*, 85–6.

That this happened in Germany, where medical research had always been presented, on both sides of the Atlantic, as less rigorously moral or only loosely guided by sympathy, was perhaps not surprising to some. But it was compounded by cases much more close to home, especially in the USA.

From early on in the American defence, there had been awkward cases. Wentworth had caused a headache in Massachusetts, and Noguchi's luetin experiments offered ripe ammunition for antivivisectionists, in a context where cases like Neisser's were exploited as more evidence of a general rot at the heart of scientific morals. But the establishment felt it could always fall back on sincere statements of their own private ethics, personal character and established practices of humanity in the laboratory. Wentworth's research quietly went away. Neisser was German. Antivivisectionist claims that Noguchi was inoculating children with syphilis could be justifiably denied. In early 1916, Udo Wile would threaten to shatter all of this.

Simon Flexner was away in China when Wile's paper came in for consideration for publication in the *Journal of Experimental Medicine*. It was published without Flexner's oversight, which would become a point of severe regret. Wile's paper, on 'Experimental Syphilis in the Rabbit Produced by the Brain Substance of the Living Paretic' was based on research undertaken by Wile that involved the removal of brain matter from non-consenting patients at the Pontiac State Hospital.[12] His methods involved a dental drill and a trocar needle, and were based on research he had seen carried out in Germany. The old spectre still threatened.[13] It was seized upon by antivivisectionists and it caught the establishment off guard.

In April, Henry James Jr would write Cannon from the Rockefeller, acknowledging that the case was 'plain as day. Wile should not have performed the operation that he has reported, and it is a great pity from our point of view that the experiment was reported in the J.E.M.'. In his view, Cannon, Keen, Lee, Welch and Flexner had to stick to their arguments and not 'hush up the attacks on Wile'. This meant condemning Wile, but put the Rockefeller men in a difficult position, since the publication had appeared in what was, effectively, the house journal. James noted that 'many medical men are really in danger of supposing that any harmless operation on a patient is justifiable if performed with a scientific purpose, even though the patient doesn't consent. I have heard this argued by most reputable and high-minded M.D's, but of course this view is one which is directly contrary

[12] Udo Wile, 'Experimental Syphilis in the Rabbit Produced by the Brain Substance of the Living Paretic', *Journal of Experimental Medicine*, 23 (1916): 199–202.
[13] The case is outlined in Lederer, *Subjected to Science*, 95–100.

to the law'.[14] All the while that the defence of experimental medicine had been focused on extolling the humanity of laboratory work, had they really lost sight of the potential for the abuse of humans in clinical settings?

Cannon admitted to Flexner that he did 'not feel competent' to judge the methods employed in the clinic, confronting an experiential limitation of 'laboratory men' and the risk that the experimental culture might be going beyond their ken.[15] To Lee, Cannon expressed a misgiving – a misgiving that had long been central to antivivisectionist arguments – that 'there was in this present flush of interest in clinical research, a danger of young men just entering upon it losing their balance and coming so interested in the pursuit of new knowledge that they forget their primary duty is to serve the welfare of the person who has committed himself to their care'.[16] He had also noted a 'grave difference of opinion' among the medical community, with hospital men in New York expressing 'hearty approval' of Wile's methods. How could they actively condemn when, unlike in their whole campaign to that point, such a condemnation only amounted to the 'feelings of these few persons' and could not be said to account for medical opinion more broadly? The community, he thought, had to formally establish 'the limit beyond which action becomes unjustifiable', noting that it was 'obvious that this limit is not now clearly defined in the minds of young men who are interested in clinical research'.[17] Meanwhile, Flexner wrote to Cannon that 'we laboratory men do not wholly appreciate the point of view and the problems of the clinicians. I should not feel competent to act for them, and I doubt whether other pure laboratory men are really able to do so'.[18] And Lee wrote to Keen that 'It is not altogether, in my mind, yet clear as to the lines along which it would be proper to perform experiments and what criteria should decide whether an individual experiment were to be performed or not. But individual consent as an invariable condition seems to me unwise and unnecessary.'[19]

Two generations of rehearsal of the arguments in favour of medical experimentation seemed to be at stake and, at the key moment, the leaders

[14] James to Cannon, 24 April 1916, Lee Papers, Box 1, Folder 31, Augustus C. Long Health Sciences Library, Columbia University, New York (CU).

[15] Cannon to Flexner, 7 June 1916, Reel 20, FA746, Series 1 Simon Flexner Paper; Subseries 1.2 Rockefeller Institute for Medical Research, Simon Flexner Papers (American Philosophical Society), RAC.

[16] Cannon to Lee, 5 June 1916, Lee Papers, Box 1, Folder 31, Augustus C. Long Health Sciences Library, Columbia University, New York (CU).

[17] Cannon to Lee, 12 May 1916, Lee Papers, Box 1, Folder 31, Augustus C. Long Health Sciences Library, Columbia University, New York (CU).

[18] Flexner to Cannon, 6 June 1916, Reel 20, FA746, Series 1 Simon Flexner Paper; Subseries 1.2 Rockefeller Institute for Medical Research, Simon Flexner Papers (American Philosophical Society), RAC.

[19] Lee to Keen, 19 May 1916, Lee Papers, Box 1, Folder 31, Augustus C. Long Health Sciences Library, Columbia University, New York (CU).

of the defence declared themselves – not out in the open, but privately to each other – unable to determine the ethics of experiment outside of laboratory conditions, or the freedom with which humans might be used by clinical researchers. While both Cannon and Flexner thought Wile was wrong, taking the matter in the abstract they cast doubt on their abilities to judge. Cannon and Keen would both publicly address their concerns about the kind of experimentation exemplified by Wile, and Cannon would push the AMA to revise its code of ethics to include consent.[20] But the public statements were watered down in a process of revision among peers and made indirect. Keen had been concerned that his need to protest openly against Wile might 'hamper research' or give the antivivisectionists ammunition to use against them at a later date and his colleagues had duly obliged in taking the sting out of his attack on Wile and re-focusing his protest towards antivivisection.[21] Cannon's push to immediately amend the ethical code did not succeed.[22] A question had been posed of medical experimentation upon which the chief experimenters could not agree an answer.

When up-and-coming men such as Francis Peabody (1881–1927) (who had also gained experience in Germany before becoming Associate Professor at Harvard Medical School) naively parroted back to Cannon his own long-rehearsed argument about trusting in the character and judgement of the best men, it suddenly rang hollow in Cannon's ears. Deeply held convictions that had been coupled with lived experience of experimental life were, it seemed, being spun into empty rhetoric or, worse, corrupted by men who truly had lost a grip on humanity, while perceiving it to be firmly within their grasp. Peabody had said that there were 'certain types of work in which it will always be difficult to decide whether they are proper or not' and that 'the future of clinical investigation will depend less on written rules and limitations, than on the type of man who is doing the work'. 'Fortunately', he added, 'it is generally true that the only men who interest themselves seriously enough in scientific medicine to be willing to give the time and attention that is required by investigation are usually among the more high-minded of the profession'.[23]

Cannon looked around at some of the young bloods in clinical research and demurred.

---

[20] W. W. Keen, 'The Inveracities of Antivivisection', *Journal of the American Medical Association*, 67 (1916): 1390–91; W. B. Cannon, 'The Right and Wrong of Making Experiments on Human Beings', *Journal of the American Medical Association*, 67 (1916): 1372–3.

[21] Keen to Lee, 8 May 1916, Lee Papers, Box 1, Folder 31, Augustus C. Long Health Sciences Library, Columbia University, New York (CU).

[22] Lederer, *Subjected to Science*, 99.

[23] Peabody to Cannon, 23 May 1916, Lee Papers, Box 1, Folder 31, Augustus C. Long Health Sciences Library, Columbia University, New York (CU).

Select Bibliography

I have not, in this bibliography, reproduced every source listed in the notes but have eliminated references – such as small editorials and published letters in medical journals and individual manuscript sources – that would only make for a more confusing perusal of the primary content that forms the narrative and its argument. Instead, I simply list the journals consulted as primary sources as well as the repositories in which the main manuscript sources can be found, alongside more significant printed primary material. The list of secondary sources is, however, complete.

Abbreviations

AAMR	Association for the Advancement of Medicine by Research
CDMR	Council for the Defense of Medical Research
MRC	Medical Research Committee
PS	Physiological Society
RAC	Rockefeller Archive Center
RDS	Research Defence Society
RUR	Rockefeller University Records
WBCA	Walter B. Cannon Archive

Manuscript Sources

Addison Papers, Bodleian Library, Oxford
Association for the Advance of Medicine by Research Papers, Wellcome Library, London
Cannon Papers, Countway Library of Medicine, Harvard University, Boston
Darwin Correspondence Project, Cambridge
Lee Papers, Columbia University Library, New York
Leishman Papers, Wellcome Library, London
MRC Papers, National Archives, Kew
Physiological Society Papers, Wellcome Library, London
Research Defence Society Papers, Wellcome Library, London
Rockefeller University Records, Rockefeller Archive Center, New York

Newspapers, Magazines and Journals

Aberdeen Journal
Birmingham Gazette and Express
British Medical Journal
Collier's
Cosmopolitan
Fortnightly Review
Harper's Monthly
Harper's Weekly
Journal of Science
Leipziger Tageblatt und Anzeiger
Luton Times and Advertiser
McClure's Magazine
Nature
New York Herald
New York Times
Nineteenth Century
Nottingham Evening Post
Pall Mall Gazette
Popular Science Monthly
Puck
Spectator
The Lancet
The Times

Printed Primary Sources

Aenosch, Eusebius, *Die Vivisektion, das grosse Verbrechen des 19. Jahrhunderts* (Dresden: H. Beringer, 1899).

American Humane Association, *Human Vivisection: A Statement and an Inquiry*, 3rd edn (Fall River, MA: American Humane Association, 1900).

Bain, Alexander, *Emotions and the Will*, 3rd edn (London: Longmans, Green, 1875).

Bishop of Ely, *Humanity and Science* (London: Research Defence Society, 1910).

Bowditch, Henry Pickering, 'The Advancement of Medicine by Research', *Science*, 4 (1896).

Bruce, David, *The Extinction of Malta Fever (A Lesson in the Use of Animal Experimentation)* (London: Macmillan, 1908).

Burdon Sanderson, John, ed., *Handbook for the Physiological Laboratory*, by E. Klein, John Burdon Sanderson, Michael Foster and Thomas Lauder Brunton, 2 vols (London: J & A Churchill, 1873).

Burdon Sanderson, Lady, *Sir John Burdon Sanderson: A Memoir* (Oxford: Clarendon Press, 1911).

Cannon, Walter B., *Animal Experimentation and Its Benefit to Mankind* (Chicago: American Medical Association, 1912).

Cannon, Walter B., 'Medical Control of Vivisection', *North American Review*, 191 ·
(1910): 814–21.

Cannon, Walter B., 'The Right and Wrong of Making Experiments on
Human Beings', *Journal of the American Medical Association*, 67 (1916):
1372–3.

Cannon, Walter B., *Some Characteristics of Antivivisection Literature* (Chicago:
American Medical Association, 1911).

Cannon, Walter B., *The Way of an Investigator: A Scientist's Experiences in Medical
Research* (New York: W. W. Norton, 1945).

Churchman, John W., 'The Value of Animal Experimentation as Illustrated by
Recent Advances in the Study of Syphilis' (Chicago: American Medical
Association, 1911).

Clover, George F., *Animal Experimentation as Viewed by the Superintendent of
a Hospital* (New York: Medical Society of the State of New York, 1909).

Curtis, John G., *Why Are Special Laws to Restrict Animal Experimentation Unwise?*
(New York: Medical Society of the State of New York, 1909).

Cushny, A. R., 'Vivisecton and Medicine: Have Experiments on Animals
Advanced Therapeutics' (1908).

Dana, Charles L., *The Service of Animal Experimentation to the Knowledge and
Treatment of Nervous Diseases* (New York: Medical Society of the State of
New York, 1909).

Darwin, Charles, *The Descent of Man* (London: John Murray, 1871).

Darwin, Francis, ed., *The Life and Letters of Charles Darwin*, 3 vols (London: John
Murray, 1887).

Darwin, Francis, and A. C. Seward, eds, *More Letters of Charles Darwin* (London:
John Murray, 1903).

Dewey, John, *The Ethics of Animal Experimentation* (New York: Medical Society of
the State of New York, 1909).

Dunn, Charles Hunter, *Animal Experimentation in Relation to Epidemic
Cerebrospinal Meningitis* (Chicago: AMA, 1911).

Eliot, Charles W., 'Animal Experimentation', in *Animal Experimentation: A Series
of Statements Indicating Its Value to Biological and Medical Science*, ed. Harold
C. Ernst, 1–3 (Boston: Little, Brown, 1902).

Ernst, Harold C., ed., *Animal Experimentation: A Series of Statements Indicating Its
Value to Biological and Medical Science* (Boston: Little, Brown, 1902).

Ewing, James, *Animal Experimentation and Cancer* (New York: Medical Society of
the State of New York, 1908).

Ferrier, David, 'The Croonian Lecture – Experiments on the Brain of Monkeys'
[read by John Burdon Sanderson], *Philosophical Transactions of the Royal Society
of London*, 165 (1875): 433–88.

Flexner, Simon, *Animal Experimentation and Infectious Diseases* (New York:
Medical Society of the State of New York, 1908).

Flexner, Simon, *The So-Called 'Affidavits Concerning the Atrocities of
Vivisection': A Refutation*. Pamphlet, reprinted from *New York Times*
(17 January 1910).

Foerster, Paul, *Die Vivisektion, die wissenschaftliche Tierfolter* (Munich:
Kupferschmid, 1913).

Foerster, Paul, *Die Vivisektion: ein Wort zur Verständigung und Mahnung, gerichtet an die vom 17. bis 24. Juli in Paris versammelten Vertreter des Tierschutzes von Dr. Paul Förster* (Berlin: Tierschutz-Verein in Comm., 1900).

Gay, Frederick P., *Immunology: A Medical Science Developed through Animal Experimentation* (Chicago: AMA, 1910).

Goltz, Friedrich, *Wider die Humanaster. Rechtfertigung eines Vivisektors* (Strassburg: Hansard, 1883).

Harnack, Erich, *Tierschutz und Vivisektion* (Berlin: Hüpeden & Merzyn, 1906).

Hatcher, Robert A., *Animal Experimentation and the Actions of Drugs* (New York: Medical Society of the State of New York, 1909)

Heidenhain, Rudolf, *Die Vivisection im Dienste der Heilkunde*, 2nd edn (Leipzig, 1879).

Hendrick, Burton J., 'American Contributions to Medical Science', *Harper's Monthly*, 129 (1914): 25–32.

Hendrick, Burton J., 'Conquering Spinal Meningitis: What the Rockefeller Institute Has Done for Children', *McClure's Magazine*, 32 (1909): 594–604.

Hendrick, Burton J., 'Work at the Rockefeller Institute: The Transplanting of Animal Organs', *McClure's Magazine*, 32 (1909): 367–83.

Hermann, L., *Die Vivisectionsfrage. Für das grössere Publicum beleuchtet* (Leipzig: F. C. W. Vogel, 1877).

Hodge, C. F., 'The Vivisection Question'. Reprinted from *Appleton's Popular Science Monthly* (September/October 1896).

Huxley, Julian, 'The Tissue-Culture King', *Cornhill Magazine*, new series 60 (1926): 422–58.

Huxley, Leonard, ed., *Life and Letters of Thomas Henry Huxley*, 2nd edn, 3 vols (London: Macmillan, 1913).

Huxley, T. H., *Collected Essays* (London: Macmillan, 1894).

Huxley, T. H., *Method and Results: Essays* (New York: D. Appleton, 1898).

Iatros [Ernst Grysanowski], *Die Vivisektion, ihr wissenschaftlicher Wert und ihre ethische Berechtigung* (Leipzig, 1877).

Keen, W. W., *Animal Experimentation and Medical Progress* (Boston: Houghton Mifflin, 1914).

Keen, W. W., *The Influence of Antivivisection on Character* (Chicago: AMA, 1912).

Keen, W. W., 'The Inveracities of Antivivisection', *Journal of the American Medical Association*, 67 (1916): 1390–91.

Keen, W. W., 'Recent Surgical Progress: A Result Chiefly of Experimental Research', *Harper's Monthly*, 118 (1909): 764–73

Kirchwey, George W., *The Legal Aspect of Animal Experimentation in the State of New York* (New York: Medical Society of the State of New York, 1909).

Laab, Artur, *Fort mit der Vivisektion! Fort mit den experimentellen Mißbräuchen and lebenden Menschen und Tieren!; Ein ernster Mahnruf und die Menschheit* (Graz: Verl. des Bundes gegen die Vivisektion in Österreich, 1905).

Lee, F. S., *The Publications of the New York Anti-Vivisection Society* (New York: Medical Society of the State of New York, 1909).

Lee, F. S., 'The Role of Experiment in Medicine: The Public and the Medical Profession', in *Scientific Features of Modern Medicine*, 154–76 (New York: Columbia University Press, 1911).

Lee, F. S., *The Sense of Pain in Man and the Lower Animals* (New York: Medical Society of the State of New York, 1908).

Lubarsch, Otto, *Über die sogenannte Vivisektion* (Halle: C. Marhold, 1905).

Ludwig, C., 'Die "Vivisection" vor dem Richterstuhl der Gegenwart: Ein Wort zur Vermittelung', *Die Gartenlaube* (1879): 417–19.

Lusk, Graham, *Animal Experimentation and Diabetes* (New York: Medical Society of the State of New York, 1909).

Mac Cormac, William, ed., *Transactions of the International Medical Congress* (London, J. W. Kolckmann, 1881).

Meltzer, S. J., *The Function of the Thyroid Glands: An Important Chapter in Modern Medicine Based upon Animal Experimentation* (New York: Medical Society of the State of New York, 1909).

Mendel, Lafayette B., *Animal Experimentation and Nutrition* (New York: Medical Society of the State of New York, 1909).

Milena, Elpis [Marie-Espérance von Schwartz], *Gemma oder Tugend and Laster* (Franz, 1877).

Moore, Veranus A., *The Relation of Animal Experimentation to the Live Stock Industry* (New York: Medical Society of the State of New York, 1909).

Oeffentliche Disputation über die Vivisektion, gehalten im Physiologischen Institute der Universität Bern am 31. Januar 1903: Nebst einem Vorwort (Dresden: Internat. Ver. z. Bekämpfung d. wiss. Tierfolter, 1904).

Official Circular Addressed to the German Universities by the Minister of Public Instruction Enjoining Safeguards against Abuses of Vivisection, with an Appendix Containing the Statements of the Several Medical Faculties (London: J. W. Kolckmann, 1885).

Paget, James, Richard Owen and Samuel Wilks, 'Vivisection: Its Pains and Its Uses', *Nineteenth Century*, 10 (1881): 902–48.

Paget, Stephen, *Experiments on Animals* (London: T. Fisher Unwin, 1900).

Paget, Stephen, ed., *For and Against Experiments on Animals: Evidence before the Royal Commission on Vivisection* (London: H. K. Lewis, 1912).

Park, William H., 'Animal Experimentation and Diphtheria' (1909).

Philanthropos [Gerald Yeo], *Physiological Cruelty: or, Fact v. Fancy. An Inquiry into the Vivisection Question* (London: Tinsley Bros., 1883).

Research Defence Society, *Evidence of Lord Justice Fletcher Moulton before the Royal Commission on Vivisection* (London: Macmillan, 1908).

Romanes, E., *The Life and Letters of George John Romanes*, New edn (London: Longmans, Green, 1896).

Rutherford, William, 'The Chief Medical Schools of the Continent', *Edinburgh Medical Journal*, 11 (1865): 341–47.

Schurman, Jacob Gould, *President Schurman on Animal Experimentation* (New York: Medical Society of the State of New York, 1909).

Simon, John, 'An Address Delivered at the Opening of the Section of Public Medicine', *British Medical Journal* (August 6, 1881): 219–23.

Simon, John, *English Sanitary Institutions*, 2nd edn (London: John Murray, 1897).

Spencer, Herbert, *Principles of Psychology* (1899; Osnabrück: Otto Zeller, 1966).

Stenz, Hermann, *Die Vivisektion, der wissenschaftliche Wahnsinn unserer Zeit: kurze Darlegung der Unhaltbarkeit, Verwerflichkeit und allgemeinen Schädlichkeit, sowie die Entbehrlichkeit des Folterns lebender Tiere zu wissenschaftlichen Zwecken* (Dresden: Weltbund gegen d. Vivisektion, 1900).

Trudeau, Edward L., *Animal Experimentation and Tuberculosis* (New York: Medical Society of the State of New York, 1909).

UK Parliament, Appendix to the First Report of the Commissioners, C. 3326 (1907).

UK Parliament, Appendix to the Fourth Report of the Commissioners, C. 3955 (1908).

UK Parliament, Appendix to the Third Report of the Commissioners, C. 3757 (1907).

UK Parliament, Final Report of the Departmental Committee on Tuberculosis, C. 6641 (1913).

UK Parliament, Final Report of the Royal Commission Appointed to Inquire into the Relation of Human and Animal Tuberculosis, C. 5761 (1911).

UK Parliament, Report of the Royal Commission on the Practice of Subjecting Live Animals to Experiments for Scientific Purposes, C. 1397 (1876).

US Government, *Vivisection: Hearing before the Senate Committee on the District of Columbia, February 21, 1900, on the Bill (S. 34) for the Further Prevention of Cruelty to Animals in the District of Columbia* (Washington, DC: Government Printing Office, 1900).

Weber, Ernst, von, *Die Folterkammern der Wissenschaft. Eine Sammlung von Thatsachen für das Laien-Publikum* (Berlin, 1879).

Welch, W. H., 'The Interdependence of Medicine and Other Sciences of Nature', in *Papers and Addresses*, 3:315–33 (Baltimore: Johns Hopkins University Press, 1920).

Welch, William H., 'On Some of the Humane Aspects of Medical Science', in *Papers and Addresses*, 3:3–8 (Baltimore: Johns Hopkins University Press, 1920).

Wells, H. G., *The Island of Dr Moreau* (London: Heinemann, 1896).

Wilde, Oscar, *The Picture of Dorian Gray* (1891; New York: Mondial, 2015).

Wile, Udo, 'Experimental Syphilis in the Rabbit Produced by the Brain Substance of the Living Paretic', *Journal of Experimental Medicine*, 23 (1916): 199–202.

Wolf, Richard, *Mensch, Tier und Vivisektion* (Leipzig: Altmann, [1900]).

Secondary Sources

Arluke, Arnold, and Boria Sax, 'Understanding Nazi Animal Protection and the Holocaust', *Anthrozoös*, 5 (1992): 6–31.

Asdal, Kristin, 'Subjected to Parliament: The Laboratory of Experimental Medicine and the Animal Body', *Social Studies of Science*, 38 (2008): 899–917.

Atalic, Bruno, and Stella Fatovic-Ferencic, 'Emanuel Edward Klein – The Father of British Microbiology and the Case of the Animal Vivisection Controversy of 1875', *Toxicologic Pathology*, 37 (2009): 708–13.

Barton, Ruth, 'Men of Science: Language, Identity and Professionalization in the Mid-Victorian Scientific Community', *History of Science*, 41:1 (2003): 73–119.

Bates, A. W. H., *Anti-Vivisection and the Profession of Medicine in Britain* (London: Palgrave, 2017).

Beers, Diane L., *For the Prevention of Cruelty: The History and Legacy of Animal Rights Activism in the United States* (Ohio: Swallow Press, 2006).

Bellon, Richard, 'Joseph Dalton Hooker's Ideals for a Professional Man of Science', *Journal of the History of Biology*, 34:1 (2001): 73–119.

Benison, Saul, 'Simon Flexner: The Evolution of a Career in Medical Science,' *Institute to University*.

Berkowitz, Carin, 'Disputed Discovery: Vivisection and Experiment in the 19th Century', *Endeavour*, 30 (2006): 98–102.

Beromeu-Sánchez, José Ramón, 'Animal Experiments, Vital Forces and Courtrooms: Mateu Orfila, François Magendie and the Study of Poisons in Nineteenth-Century France', *Annals of Science*, 69 (2012): 1–26.

Bittel, Carla, 'Science, Suffrage, and Experimentation: Mary Putnam Jacobi and the Controversy over Vivisection in Late Nineteenth-Century America', *Bulletin of the History of Medicine*, 79 (2005): 664–94.

Bliss, Michael, *William Osler: A Life in Medicine* (Oxford: Oxford University Press, 2007).

Boddice, Rob, *A History of Attitudes and Behaviours toward Animals in Eighteenth- and Nineteenth-Century Britain: Anthropocentrism and the Emergence of Animals* (Lewiston: Mellen, 2009).

Boddice, Rob, *A History of Feelings* (London: Reaktion, 2019).

Boddice, Rob, 'Bestiality in a Time of Smallpox: Dr Jenner and the "Modern Chimera"', in *Exploring Animal Encounters: Philosophical, Cultural and Historical Perspectives*, ed. Dominik Ohrem and Matthew Calarco, 155–78 (London: Palgrave, 2018).

Boddice, Rob, 'The End of Anthropocentrism', in *Anthropocentrism: Humans, Animals, Environments*, ed. Rob Boddice, 1–18 (Leiden: Brill, 2011).

Boddice, Rob, 'German Methods, English Morals: Physiological Networks and the Question of Callousness, c.1870–1881', in *Anglo-German Scholarly Relations in the Long Nineteenth Century*, ed. Heather Ellis and Ulrike Kirchberger, 84–102 (Leiden: Brill, 2014).

Boddice, Rob, 'The Historical Animal Mind: "Sagacity" in Nineteenth-Century Britain', in *Experiencing Animals: Encounters between Animal and Human Minds*, ed. Robert W. Mitchell and Julie Smith, 65–78 (New York: Columbia University Press, 2012).

Boddice, Rob, *The History of Emotions* (Manchester: Manchester University Press, 2018).

Boddice, Rob, 'The Moral Status of Animals and the Historical Human Cachet', *JAC: A Journal of Rhetoric, Culture and Politics*, 30:3–4 (2010): 457–89.

Boddice, Rob, *The Science of Sympathy: Morality, Evolution and Victorian Civilization* (Urbana-Champaign: University of Illinois Press, 2016).

Boddice, Rob, 'Species of Compassion: Aesthetics, Anaesthetics and Pain in the Physiological Laboratory', *19: Interdisciplinary Studies in the Long Nineteenth Century*, 15 (2012).

Boddice, Rob, 'Vivisecting Major: A Victorian Gentleman Scientist Defends Animal Experimentation, 1876–1885', *Isis*, 102 (2011): 215–37.

Boddice, Rob, and Mark Smith, *Emotion, Sense, Experience* (Cambridge: Cambridge University Press, 2020).

Bourke, Joanna, *The Story of Pain: From Prayer to Painkillers* (Oxford: Oxford University Press, 2014).

Bourke, Joanna, *What It Means to Be Human: Reflections from 1791 to the Present* (London: Virago, 2011).

Bowler, Peter J., 'Lankester, Sir (Edwin) Ray (1847–1929)', in *Oxford Dictionary of National Biography* (Oxford: Oxford University Press, 2004).

Bretschneider, H., *Der Streit um die Vivisektion im 19. Jahrhundert. Verlauf – Argumente – Ergebnisse* (Stuttgart, 1962).

Brock,D. Heyward, 'The Doctor as Dramatic Hero', *Perspectives in Biology and Medicine*, 34 (1991): 279–95.

Bryder, Linda, 'Tuberculosis and the MRC', in *Historical Perspectives on the Role of the MRC: Essays in the History of the Medical Research Council of the United Kingdom and Its Predecessor, the Medical Research Committee, 1913–1953*, ed. Joan Austoker and Linda Bryder, 1–21 (Oxford: Oxford University Press, 1989).

Buettinger, Craig, 'Antivivisection and the Charge of Zoophil-Psychosis in the Early Twentieth Century', *The Historian*, 55 (1992): 277–88.

Buettinger, Craig, 'Women and Antivivisection in Late Nineteenth-Century America', *Journal of Social History*, 30 (1997): 857–72.

Butler, Stella V. F., 'Centers and Peripheries: The Development of British Physiology, 1870–1914', *Journal of the History of Biology*, 21 (1988): 473–500.

Catlet, Stephen, 'Huxley, Hutton and the "White Rage": A Debate on Vivisection at the Metaphysical Society', *Archives of Natural History*, 11 (1983): 181–9.

Colby, Robert A., ' "How It Strikes a Contemporary": The "Spectator" as Critic', *Nineteenth-Century Fiction*, 11 (1956): 182–206.

Corner, George W., *A History of the Rockefeller Institute 1901–1953, Origins and Growth* (New York: Rockefeller Institute Press, 1964).

Cunningham, Andrew, and Perry Williams, eds, *The Laboratory Revolution in Medicine* (Cambridge: Cambridge University Press, 1992).

Cushing, Harvey, *The Life of Sir William Osler* (Oxford, 1940).

Daston, Lorraine, and Peter Galison, *Objectivity* (New York: Zone Books, 2007).

Davis, John, 'Higher Education Reform and the German Model: A Victorian Discourse', in *Anglo-German Scholarly Relations in the Long Nineteenth Century*, ed. Heather Ellis and Ulrike Kirchberger, 39–62 (Leiden: Brill, 2014).

Dror, Otniel, 'The Affect of Experiment: The Turn to Emotions in Anglo-American Physiology, 1900–1940', *Isis*, 90 (1999): 205–37.

Elston, Mary Ann, 'The Anti-Vivisectionist Movement and the Science of Medicine', in *Challenging Medicine*, ed. Jonathan Gabe, David Kelleher and Gareth Williams, 160–80 (London: Routledge, 1994).

Elston, Mary Ann, 'Women and Anti-Vivisection in Victorian England, 1870–1900', in *Vivisection in Historical Perspective*, ed. Nicolaas A. Rupke, 259–94 (London: Croom Helm, 1987).

Flexner, James Thomas, *An American Saga: The Story of Helen Thomas and Simon Flexner* (New York: Fordham University Press, 1993).

French, Richard D., *Antivivisection and Medical Science in Victorian Society* (Princeton, NJ: Princeton University Press, 1975).

Friedman, David M., *The Immortalists; Charles Lindbergh, Dr. Alexis Carrel, and Their Daring Quest to Live Forever* (New York: Harper, 2007).

Fye, W. Bruce, 'Carl Ludwig and the Leipzig Physiological Institute: "A Factory of New Knowledge"', *Circulation*, 74 (1986): 920–28.

Fye, W. Bruce, *The Development of American Physiology: Scientific Medicine in the Nineteenth Century* (Baltimore: Johns Hopkins University Press, 1987).

Geison, Gerald L., *Michael Foster and the Cambridge School of Physiology: The Scientific Enterprise in Late Victorian Society* (Princeton, NJ: Princeton University Press, 1978).

Gere, Cathy, *Pain, Pleasure, and the Greater Good: From the Panopticon to the Skinner Box and Beyond* (Chicago: University of Chicago Press, 2017).

Geroulanos, Stephanos, and Todd Meyers, *The Human Body in the Age of Catastrophe: Brittleness, Integration, Science, and the Great War* (Chicago: University of Chicago Press, 2018).

Gest, Howard, 'Dr. Martin Arrowsmith: Scientist and Medical Hero', *Perspectives in Biology and Medicine*, 35 (1991): 116–24.

Gill, Rebecca, *Calculating Compassion: Humanity and Relief in War, Britain, 1870–1914* (Manchester: Manchester University Press, 2013).

Gollin, Alfred M., *The Observer and J. L. Garvin, 1908–1914* (Oxford: Oxford University Press, 1960).

Goodman, Jordan, and Anthony McElligot, eds, *Useful Bodies: Humans in the Service of Medical Science in the Twentieth Century* (Baltimore: Johns Hopkins University Press, 2003).

Gossel, Patricia Peck, 'William Henry Welch and the Antivivisection Legislation in the District of Columbia, 1896–1900', *Journal of the History of Medicine and Allied Sciences*, 40 (1985): 397–419.

Gradmann, Christoph, ' "It Seemed about Time to Try One of Those Modern Medicines": Animal and Human Experimentation in the Chemotherapy of Sleeping Sickness 1905–1908', in *Twentieth Century Ethics of Human Subjects Research: Historical Perspectives on Values, Practices, and Regulations*, ed. Volker Roelcke, 83–97 (Stuttgart: Franz Steiner, 2004).

Guarnieri, Patrizia, 'Moritz Schiff (1823–96): Experimental Physiology and Noble Sentiment in Florence', in *Vivisection in Historical Perspective*, ed. Nicolaas A. Rupke, 105–24 (London: Croom Helm, 1987).

Halttunen, Karen, 'Humanitarianism and the Pornography of Pain in Anglo-American Culture', *American Historical Review*, 100 (1995): 303–34.

Halverson, Kristin, 'Physiological Cruelty? Discussing and Developing Vivisection in Great Britain, 1875–1901', MA thesis, Södertörn University (2016).

Hamilton, Susan, 'Reading and the Popular Critique of Science in the Victorian Anti-Vivisection Press: Frances Power Cobbe's Writing for the Victoria Street Society', *Victorian Review*, 36 (2010): 66–79.

Hansen, Bert, 'Medical History for the Masses: How American Comic Books Celebrated Heroes of Medicine in the 1940s', *Bulletin of the History of Medicine*, 78 (2004): 148–91.

Hanson, Elizabeth, 'Women Scientists at the Rockefeller Institute, 1901–1940', in *Creating a Tradition of Biomedical Research: Contributions to the History of the Rockefeller University*, ed. Darwin H. Stapleton, 211–25 (New York: Rockefeller University Press, 2004).

Haskell, Thomas L., 'Capitalism and the Origins of the Humanitarian Sensibility', parts I and II, *American Historical Review*, 90 (1985): 339–61, 547–66.

Hochschild, Arlie Russel, *The Managed Heart: Commercialization of Human Feeling* (Berkeley: University of California Press, 1983).

Honigsbaum, Frank, 'Christopher Addison: A Realist in Pursuit of Dreams', in *Doctors, Politics and Society: Historical Essays*, ed. Dorothy Porter and Roy Porter, 229–46 (Amsterdam: Rodopi, 1993).

Hornsby, Asha, 'Unfeeling Brutes? The 1875 Royal Commission on Vivisection and the Science of Suffering', *Victorian Review*, 45 (2019): 97–115.

Hutchison, John, *Champions of Charity: War and the Rise of the Red Cross* (Boulder, CO: Westview Press, 1996).

Institute to University: A Seventy-Fifth Anniversary Colloquium, June 8, 1976 (New York: Rockefeller University, 1976).

'John C. Dalton, Jr. (1825–1889) Experimental Physiologist', *Journal of the American Medical Association*, 203 (1968): 221–22.

Kean, Hilda, ' "The Smooth Cool Men of Science": The Feminist and Socialist Response to Vivisection', *History Workshop Journal*, 40 (1995): 16–38.

Lambert, R., *Sir John Simon, 1816–1904 and English Social Administration* (London: MacGibbon & Kee, 1963).

Landecker, Hannah, *Culturing Life: How Cells Became Technologies* (Cambridge, MA: Harvard University Press, 2007).

Landsborough Thomson, A., 'Origin of the British Legislative Provision for Medical Research', *Journal of Social Policy*, 2 (1973): 41–54.

Lansbury, Coral, *The Old Brown Dog: Women, Workers and Vivisection in Edwardian England* (Madison: University of Wisconsin Press, 1985).

Lederer, Susan, 'The Controversy over Animal Experimentation in America, 1880–1914', in *Vivisection in Historical Perspective*, ed. Nicolaas Rupke, 236–58 (London: Croom Helm, 1987).

Lederer, Susan, 'Hideyo Noguchi's Luetin Experiment and the Antivivisectionists', *Isis*, 76 (1985): 31–48.

Lederer, Susan, 'Orphans as Guinea Pigs: American Children and Medical Experimenters, 1890–1930', in *In the Name of the Child: Health and Welfare, 1880–1940*, ed. Roger Cooter, 96–123 (New York: Routledge, 2013).

Lederer, Susan, 'Political Animals: The Shaping of Biomedical Research Literature in Twentieth-Century America', *Isis*, 83 (1992): 61–79.

Lederer, Susan, *Subjected to Science: Human Experimentation in America before the Second World War* (Baltimore: Johns Hopkins University Press, 1995).

Lemov, Rebecca, *World as Laboratory: Experiments with Mice, Mazes, and Men* (New York: Hill and Wang, 2006).

Leroy, Gaylord C., 'Richard Holt Hutton', *PMLA*, 56 (1941): 809–40.

Libell, Monica, *Morality beyond Humanity: Schopenhauer, Grysanowski, and Schweitzer on Animal Ethics* (Lund, 2001).

Loveridge, Ann, 'Historical, Fictional and Illustrative Readings of the Vivisected Body 1873–1913', doctoral thesis, Canterbury Christ Church University (2017).

Lyons, Dan, 'Protecting Animals versus the Pursuit of Knowledge: The Evolution of the British Animal Research Policy Process', *Society & Animals*, 19 (2011): 356–67.

MacNalty, Arthur Salusbury, *Sir William Collins, Surgeon and Statesman* (London: Chadwick Trust, 1949).

Maehle, Andreas Holger, *Doctors, Honour and the Law: Medical Ethics in Imperial Germany* (Houndmills, UK: Palgrave, 2009).

Maehle, Andreas-Holger, 'The Ethical Discourse on Animal Experimentation, 1650–1900', in *Doctors and Ethics: The Earlier Historical Setting of Professional Ethics*, ed. A. Wear, J. Geyer-Kordesch and R. French, 203–51. The Wellcome Series in the History of Medicine, Clio Medica, vol. 24 (Amsterdam, 1993).

Maehle, Andreas-Holger, 'Organisierte Tierversuchsgegner: Gründe und Grenzen ihrer gesellschaftlichen Wirkung, 1879–1933', in *Medizinkritische Bewegungen im Deutschen Reich (ca. 1870–ca. 1933)*, ed. M. Dinges, 109–25. Medizin, Gesellschaft und Geschichte suppl. vol. 9 (Stuttgart, 1996).

Mayer, Jed, 'The Expression of the Emotions in Man and Laboratory Animals', *Victorian Studies*, 50:3 (2008): 399–417.

McKellar, Shelley, 'Innovation in Modern Surgery: Alexis Carrel and Blood Vessel Repair', in *Creating a Tradition of Biomedical Research: Contributions to the History of the Rockefeller University*, ed. Darwin H. Stapleton, 131–50 (New York: Rockefeller University Press, 2004).

Mckibbin, Ross, 'Politics and the Medical Hero: A.J. Cronin's *The Citadel*', *English Historical Review*, 123 (2008): 651–78.

Miller, Ian, 'Necessary Torture? Vivisection, Suffragette Force-Feeding, and Responses to Scientific Medicine in Britain c. 1870–1920', *Journal of the History of Medicine and Allied Sciences*, 64 (2009): 333–72.

Morantz, Regina Markell, 'Feminism, Professionalism, and Germs: The Thought of Mary Putnam Jacobi and Elizabeth Blackwell', *American Quarterly*, 34 (1982): 459–78.

Morgan, K., 'Addison, Christopher, First Viscount Addison (1869–1951), Politician', in *Oxford Dictionary of National Biography* (Oxford: Oxford University Press, 2004).

Moruno, Dolores Martín, Brenda Lynn Edgar and Marie Leyder, 'Feminist Perspectives on the History of Humanitarian Relief (1870–1945)', *Medicine, Conflict and Survival*, 36 (2020): 2–18.

Neff, Roland, *Der Streit um den wissenschaftlichen Tierversuch in der Schweiz des 19. Jahrhunderts* (Basel: Schwabe, 1989).

Otis, Laura, ' "Howled out of the Country": Wilkie Collins and H.G. Wells Retry David Ferrier', in *Neurology and Literature, 1860–1920*, ed. Anne Stiles, 27–51 (Houndmills, UK: Palgrave, 2007).

Preece, Rod, 'Darwin, Christianity and the Great Vivisection Debate', *Journal of the History of Ideas*, 64 (2003): 399–419.

Richards, Stewart, 'Anaesthetics, Ethics and Aesthetics: Vivisection in the Late Nineteenth-Century British Laboratory', in *The Laboratory Revolution in Medicine*, ed. Andrew Cunningham and Perry Williams, 142–69 (Cambridge: Cambridge University Press, 1992).

Richards, Stewart, 'Drawing the Life-Blood of Physiology: Vivisection and the Physiologists' Dilemma, 1870–1900', *Annals of Science*, 43 (1986): 27–56.

Robb-Smith, A. H. T., 'Medical Education', in *The History of the University of Oxford*, ed. M. G. Brock and M. C. Curthoys, 6: 563–82 (Oxford: Clarendon Press, 1997).

Romano, Terrie M., *Making Medicine Scientific: John Burdon Sanderson and the Culture of Victorian Science* (Baltimore: Johns Hopkins University Press, 2002).

Rosenberg, Charles E., 'Martin Arrowsmith: The Scientists as Hero', *American Quarterly*, 15 (1963): 447–58.

Ross, Karen D., 'Recruiting "Friends of Medical Progress": Evolving Tactics in the Defense of Animal Experimentation, 1910s and 1920s', *Journal of the History of Medicine and Allied Sciences*, 70 (2015): 365–93.

Rupke, Nicolaas, 'Pro-Vivisection in England in the Early 1880s: Arguments and Motives', in *Vivisection in Historical Perspective*, ed. Nicolaas Rupke, 188–208 (London: Croom Helm, 1987).

Rupke, Nicolaas, ed., *Vivisection in Historical Perspective* (London: Croom Helm, 1987).

Salvatici, Silvia, *A History of Humanitarianism, 1755–1989: In the Name of Others* (Manchester: Manchester University Press, 2019).

Sauerteig, Lutz, 'Ethische Richtlinien, Patientenrechte and ärztliches Verhalten bei der Arzneimittelerprobung (1892–1931)', *Medizinhistorisches Journal*, 35 (2000): 303–34.

Sax, Boria, *Animals in the Third Reich: Pets, Scapegoats, and the Holocaust* (New York: Continuum, 2000).

Schickore, Jutta, *About Method: Experimenters, Snake Venom, and the History of Writing Scientifically* (Chicago: University of Chicago Press, 2017).

Schmidt, Ulf, *Secret Science: A Century of Poison Warfare and Human Experiments* (Oxford: Oxford University Press, 2015).

Schmidt, Ulf, and A. Frewer, eds, *History and Theory of Human Experimentation: The Declaration of Helsinki and Modern Medical Ethics* (Stuttgart: Franz Steiner, 2007).

Shmuely, Shira Dina, 'The Bureaucracy of Empathy: Vivisection and the Question of Animal Pain in Britain, 1876–1912', PhD thesis, Massachusetts Institute of Technology (2017).

Stapleton, Darwin H., ed., *Creating a Tradition of Biomedical Research: Contributions to the History of the Rockefeller University* (New York: Rockefeller University Press, 2004).

Stiles, Anne, *Popular Fiction and Brain Science in the Late Nineteenth Century* (Cambridge: Cambridge University Press, 2012).

Taithe, Bertrand, ' "Cold Calculation in the Faces of Horrors?" Pity, Compassion and the Making of Humanitarian Protocols', in *Medicine, Emotion and Disease, 1700–1950*, ed. Fay Bound Alberti, 79–99 (Houndmills, UK: Palgrave, 2006).

Taithe, Bertrand, and John Borton, 'History, Memory and "Lessons Learnt" from Humanitarian Practitioners', *European Review of History: Revue européenne d'histoire*, 23 (2016): 210–24.

Takahashi, Aya, 'Hideyo Noguchi, the Pursuit of Immunity and the Persistence of Fame: A Reappraisal', in *Creating a Tradition of Biomedical Research: Contributions to the History of the Rockefeller University*, ed. Darwin H. Stapleton, 227–39 (New York: Rockefeller University Press, 2004).

Tansey, E. M., ' "The Queen Has Been Dreadfully Shocked": Aspects of Teaching Experimental Physiology Using Animals in Britain, 1876–1986', *Advances in Physiology Education*, 19 (1998): 18–33.

Tansey, E. M., 'The Wellcome Physiological Research Laboratories 1894–1904: The Home Office, Pharmaceutical Firms, and Animal Experiments', *Medical History*, 33 (1989): 1–41.

Tröhler, Ulrich, and Andreas-Holger Maehle, 'Anti-Vivisection in Nineteenth-Century Germany and Switzerland: Motives and Methods', in *Vivisection in Historical Perspective*, ed. Nicolaas Rupke, 149–87 (London: Croom Helm, 1987).

Unti, Bernard, ' "The Doctors Are So Sure That They Only Are Right": The Rockefeller Institute and the Defeat of Vivisection Reform in New York, 1908–1914', in *Creating a Tradition of Biomedical Research: Contributions to the History of the Rockefeller University*, ed. Darwin H. Stapleton, 175–90 (New York: Rockefeller University Press, 2004).

Waller, J. C., 'Gentlemanly Men of Science: Sir Francis Galton and the Professionalization of the British Life-Sciences', *Journal of the History of Biology*, 34:1 (2001): 83–114.

Warner, John Harley, 'Ernst, Harold Clarence', in *American National Biography* (Oxford: Oxford University Press, 1999).

Weisz, George, *Divide and Conquer: A Comparative History of Medical Specialization* (Oxford: Oxford University Press, 2005).

Westacott, E., *A Century of Vivisection and Anti-Vivisection: A Study of Their Effect upon Science, Medicine and Human Life during the Past Hundred Years* (Ashingdon, UK: C. W. Daniel, 1949).

Westermann-Cicio, Mary L., 'Of Mice and Medical Men: The Medical Profession's Response to the Vivisection Controversy in Turn of the Century America', PhD thesis, State University of New York (2001).

Wetherby, Aelwen D., *Private Aid, Political Activism: American Medical Relief to Spain and China, 1936–1949* (Columbia: University of Missouri Press, 2017).

White, Paul S., 'Darwin Wept: Science and the Sentimental Subject', *Journal of Victorian Culture*, 16 (2011): 195–213.

White, Paul S., 'The Experimental Animal in Victorian Britain', in *Thinking with Animals: New Perspectives on Anthropomorphism*, ed. Lorraine Daston and Gregg Mitman, 59–81 (New York: Columbia University Press, 2005).

White, Paul S., 'Sympathy under the Knife: Experimentation and Emotion in Late Victorian Medicine', in *Medicine, Emotion and Disease, 1700–1950*, ed. Fay Bound Alberti, 100–24 (Houndmills, UK: Palgrave, 2006).

Willis, Martin, 'Unmasking Immorality: Popular Opposition to Laboratory Science in Late Victorian Britain', in *Repositioning Victorian Sciences: Shifting Centres in Nineteenth-Century Scientific Thinking*, ed. David Clifford, 207–18 (London: Anthem Press, 2006).

Wilson, David A. H., 'The Public Relations of Experimental Animal Psychology in Britain in the 1970s', *Contemporary British History*, 18 (2004): 27–46.

Woodfield, Malcolm, 'Victorian Weekly Reviews and Reviewing after 1860: R.H. Hutton and the *Spectator*', *Yearbook of English Studies*, 16 (1986): 74–91.

Woolsey, Thomas A., and Robert E. Burke, 'The Playwright, the Practitioner, the Politician, the President, and the Pathologist: A Guide to the 1900 Senate Document Titled "Vivisection"', *Perspectives in Biology and Medicine*, 30 (1987): 235–58.

Worboys, Michael, 'Klein, Edward Emanuel (1844–1925)', in *Oxford Dictionary of National Biography* (Oxford: Oxford University Press, 2004).

Index